WOMEN AND NUTRITION IN HIMALAYA

Women and Nutrition in Himalaya

Dr. B.R. Pant
Department of Geography
Government P.G. College
Rudrapur

ANMOL PUBLICATIONS PVT. LTD.
NEW DELHI - 110 002 (INDIA)

ANMOL PUBLICATIONS PVT. LTD.
4374/4B, Ansari Road, Daryaganj
New Delhi - 110 002
Ph.: 23261597, 23278000
Visit us at: www.anmolpublications.com

Women and Nutrition in Himalaya

First Published, 2004
ISBN 81-261-1970-5

PRINTED IN INDIA

Published by J.L. Kumar for Anmol Publications Pvt. Ltd., New Delhi - 110 002 and Printed at Mehra Offset Press, Delhi.

Contents

PREFACE

More than two billion people of the world subsist on diets deficient in essential vitamins and minerals required for normal growth and development and for the prevention of premature death and disabilities such as blindness and mental retardation. Millions suffer from diseases caused by the consumption of inadequate nutritious food and unsafe water. About 40% of women in Sub-Saharan Africa suffer from iron deficiency anemia, as against approximately 60% of women in South Africa and in India. This rises to a staggering 83% during pregnancy. Therefore the poor care of girls and women by their husbands and elders leads to higher child malnutrition.

According to the World Health Organization, health is a state of complete physical, mental and social wellbeing and not merely an absence of disease or infirmity (Jhonstone, 1994). This has opened new vista of approach and has widened the scope and expectation involved in the promotion of health. Keeping this approach in mind the health of women need to be considered in broader perspective. So the evaluation of the health and nutrition status of the women require special attention.

Generally the nutrition status of a person is closely related to food adequacy and its distribution, per capita income, female literacy, family size, type of occupation, rate of population growth, hygiene sense, environmental sanitation and access to health, education, safe drinking water and other social services while the extent of nutrition awareness forms its basic ground in particular. Nutrition deficiency means lack of resistant power against communicable, non-communicable or deficiency diseases. In this part of Himalaya, excess workload coupled with inadequate intake of nutritious food have led normal to severe mal/under-nutritional problem among the women. In fact cooking fewer meals, eating cold or leftover food or some times even skeepping meals have been reported in the several parts of the region as fuel saving strategies. This, over a period, can result a !ower nutritional level. The main aim of this study is to calculate the nutrition status of most vulnerable section of the society—women as per their stage-general (non-pregnant-non-lactating), pregnant and lactating with the support of their socio-economic background. The present study will be helpful for the policy planning to overcome this severe problem of nutrition deficiency.

The present investigation is based on the first hand information. In all 136 sample women from 14 sample villages of Uttarakhand Himalaya have been surveyed comprehensively. The present book has been divided into five chapters. The first chapter consists of research problem, review of literature, objectives, research methodology and about the study area. The second chapter is devoted to environmental and demographic profile of Indian Himalaya which is based on secondary sources. The third chapter is given to the geophysical environment of the whole region (Uttarakhand)—physiography, geology, drainage, climate, natural vegetation and soils, which are based on secondary data and personal observations. The fourth chapter, which also devotes to the whole region of Uttarakhand, consists of eco-cultural environment in which demographic profile, fairs and festivals, landuse and allied sectors, food production and nutrition availability, infrastructural development and accessibility have been discussed. The fifth chapter is on women and nutrition-a case study which is based on first hand information of 136 sample women from fourteen sample villages. This chapter includes the category-wise socio-economic structure, housing and environmental sanitation, hygiene pattern, food habits, study of Body Mass Index, food consumption, nutrients intake pattern, etc. The last chapter provides the summary and conclusions.

This work could not have seen the light of the day without the valuable help of eminent scientists. The list of the experts who assisted in this endeavour is long and dreary I wish to thank all of them.

Grateful acknowledgement is conveyed to the University Grants Commission, 35, Feroz Shah Road, New Delhi for financial assistance during the Minor Research Project (1999-2002).

I express my deep sense of gratitude to Padamsree Prof. Mohammed Shafi, Department of Geography, A.M.U., Aligarh, Mr. V. Paul I.A.S Secretary Uttaranchal Government, Prof. P. C. Barakoti, Director Higher Education Uttaranchal and Prof. C. Gopalan, Nutrition Foundation of India, New Delhi, for their inspiration and guidance. I also express my gratitude respectively to Prof. J.C. Tiwary and Prof. M. Sayal, Principals, Govt. P.G. College, Bageshwar and Rudrapur for their kind help in various ways. I must put to record to my gratefulness to my then students Mr. G.S. Rawat, Mr. Narendra Singh Rautela, Mr. Gokul Chandra Pande, Mr. Bhaskar Pant and Mr. Bhariab Giri, Govt. P.G. College Bageshwar for their kind support during field work.

I would also express my esteemed gratitude toward my wife Dr. (Smt.) Hemlata for her kind support in adverse circumstances.

I would like to express my sincere thanks to all those, in particular, members of the interviewed families who volunteered the author at various stages of this work.

Finally I thanks to Mr. K. D. Joshi of Anmol Publications Pvt. Ltd., New Delhi for publication of this manuscript with great care and patience.

Rudrapur

(B. R. Pant)

1

INTRODUCTION

1.1 The Problem

The nutrition status of the people is an important indicator of the development of a country. Despite spectacular increase in foodgrains in recent decades the problem of chronic malnutrition continues to exist extensively, especially among children and women, because they are caught in the relentless sequence of ignorance, poverty, inadequate nutritious food intake and disease. Generally the nutrition status of a person, village, region or country is closely related to food adequacy and its distribution, per capita income, female literacy, family size, type of occupation, rate of population growth, hygienic sense, environmental sanitation and access to health, education, safe drinking water, and other social services, while the extent of nutrition awareness forms its basic grounds in particular. Thus the nutrition status is a result of complex and interrelated set of determining factors.

In the beginning of the 21st century, over 840 million people of the world, mostly from Africa, South Asia, and Latin America still do not get sufficient nutritious food to meet the basic requirements for energy and protein. More than two billion people subsists on diets that lack of essential vitamins and minerals required for normal growth and development and for the prevention of premature death and disabilities such as blindness and mental retardation. Millions suffer from disease caused by the consumption of inadequate nutritious food and unsafe water. About 40% of women in Sub-Saharan Africa suffer from iron deficiency anaemia, as against to approximately 60% of women on South Africa and in India. This rises to a staggering 83% during pregnancy. Therefore, the poor care of girls and women by respectively their parents, husbands and elders leads to higher child malnutrition.

According to the World Health Organization (1948) "health is a stage of complete physical, mental and social well being and not merely an absence of disease of infirmity (Johnstone, 1994)". This has opened new vista of approach and has widened the scope and expectation involved in the promotion of health. Keeping of this approach in mind the health of women need to be considered in a broader perspective. So the evaluation of the health and nutrition status of the women require special attention.

According the 10th annual report of the Bread for the World Institute, during last fifty years, almost 400 million people died due to hunger and poor sanitation the world over. Further report says that the largest number of people who suffer nutritional deficiencies in South Asia, where poverty, discrimination against women, unsafe water and poor sanitation contribute to poor health. More than 50% of children under the age of five are stunted due to insufficient food consumption and poor health condition (Menon, N.C., *Hindustan Times,* 10-02-2000).

According to the Untied Nations Population Fund, the proportion of malnourished people has declined, but there has been an increase in the absolute number of people affected. The most affected are the women (Anon, 1998). The incidence of low birth weight babies – a sensitive indicator of well being of women has increased in nearly 50% of the countries (Hazra, 1998).

India has the highest number of female mortality during pregnancy and childbirth. According to the states of the World's Children Report, 410 out of every 1 Lakh new born babies in the country loss their mother during the delivery itself. More than 75% of the total population reside in the rural areas and slums in India. The economy of the rural people depend on agricultural practices which are mostly performed by the neglected and ignored section of the society – women; who constitute nearly 50% of the total population. Likewise India, women of Uttarakhand Himalaya also performs agricultural practices (primary activities) and contribute a major share of family economy in terms of kinds such as foodgrains, oil seeds, vegetables, fruits, milk, wool, etc.

In this part of Himalaya, excess workload coupled with inadequate intake of nutritious food have led normal to server mal/under nutritional problem among the women. Infact cooking less than required meals, eating cold or leftover food or sometimes-even skeeping meals have been reported not only in the region but also in several developing countries as fuel saving strategies. This practice over a longer period, can result lower nutritional levels.

Nutritional deficiency means lack of resistant power to protect from communicable, non-communicable or deficiency diseases. Despite overcoming the famines and eliminating classical nutritional deficiency syndromes like beri-beri, pellagra, scurvy, etc. However, the problem of protein – energy malnutrition, micro nutrients (minerals and vitamins) deficiency, deficiency of iron, vitamin A and iodine are especially important because of their serious health consequences and geographic distribution. These nutrition deficiency lead to the diseases like kwashiorkor, rickets, anaemia, blindness, goitre, etc. and even affects the learning ability. I.Q., productivity and physical and hormonal growth of human being.

The main objective of this study is to calculate the nutrition status of most vulnerable section among the people-women-as per their stage i.e. normal or general (non-lactating – non-pregnant), pregnant and lactating with the support of their socio-economic backgrounds, awareness of environmental sanitation, hygiene pattern, etc. The present investigation will through the light on the complete scenario of women and nutrition in Uttarakhand Himalaya which will certainly provide valuable direction for the policy planning to overcome this severe problem of nutritional deficiency.

1.2 Review of Literature

Women not only in the Himalaya but also in the World as a whole have generally enjoyed a lower status than men in the society. Various cultural values and social institutions are responsible for lower status of women in comparison to men in our society. Due to various vigorous women's movements in recent past there has been a considerable increase of interest in the health and nutrition problem of women in the country.

Still undeveloped branch of Geography, the work in the field of Medical Geography was carried out in 1930s. In detail, Nutrition Geography is most important branch of Medical Geography. A number of macro and micro level studies have been made in the field of health and nutrition and its related fields in recent decades. Majority of these studies are concerned to food production and nutritional status of the people. The present investigation on women and nutrition has been particularly studied by the scientists of World Health Organisation, International Food Policy Research Institute, Washington D.C.; UNICEF; National Institute Nutrition, Hyderabad; Indian Council of Medical Research, New Delhi; International Institute of Population Sciences, Mumbai; Nutrition Foundation of India, New Delhi; National Nutrition Monitoring Bureau (NNMB), the National Family Health Survey (NFHS), Department of Women and Child Development Government of India, etc.

Other individual eminent workers who have carried out directly or indirectiy on socio-economic and nutritional status surveys in different parts of the World include Kramer (1987),

Baird (1947), Barros *et al.* (1987), Simpson *et al.* (1975), Samuel and Rao (1992), Chatterjee and Lambert (1990), Kisanga (1990), Krasovec (1991), Tripathi *et al.* (1987), Karmarker *et al.* (1995), Geervani *et al.* (1983), Gopalan (1989a and 1989b), Gopalan and S. Kaur (1989), Gopalan and H. Kaur (1993), Ramotra (1989 and 1995), Sood and Nagla (1999), Wong (1995), Chaudhary and Trovoto (1994), Wong (1999), Salaff (1976), Baker (1996), Srinivasan and Kanitkar (1989), Rao (1989), Srikantia (1989), Ram Chandran (1989a , 1989b and 1996), Mathai (1989), Chatterjee (1989), Hazra (1998), Sachdeve (1997), Prentice (1998), Vir and Nigam (2001), etc. But these studies are primarily confined to other than Himalayan Region. The present attempt is basically non-clinical (geographical point of view). Therefore, the present exercise will not only fill up the academic gap but also provide the measures for nutritional security to women and children at large (Pant, 2001, 2002, 2003 and in press a, b, c).

1.3 Aims and Objectives

The issue of women and nutrition in the mountainous region like Uttarakhand Himalaya is not highly complex and intricate but also difficult. It is not possible to examine all individual women for nutritional study. Therefore, it is inevitably limited to some major aspects of limited individual women. The specific objectives of the present study are:-

1. To study the environmental degration and demographic profile of the Indian Himalaya.
2. To study the geo-physical and eco-cultural environment of the region as a whole (Uttarakhand).
3. To select the sample women – normal or general (non-lactating and non-pregnant), pregnant and lactating women from the sample villages located in different geo-physical divisions.
4. To study the socio-economic status of sample women.
5. To study the specific aspects such as fertility pattern, abortion tendency, intoxicants use and some silent

features of lactating women, pregnant women and their offsprings.

6. To study the infrastructural facilities available in the region and sample villages.
7. To study the housing and environmental sanitation condition.
8. To study the personal hygiene and dietary pattern of the sample.
9. To calculate the category-wise nutrition status of the total sample.
10. To study the awareness among the sample.
11. To suggest some feasible measures to overcome this serious burning problem.

1.4 Hypothesis

Women of this rural based country are busy since early morning to late night. Right from cleaning the agricultural fields, breaking of pods, removal of manure, fetching water from distant hilly terrain, collecting and carrying heavy loads of fuel wood, fodder, litter fall on head or back from remote places, cooking, nursing babies, washing and than feeding as well as milking animals etc. Besides these routine works women also look-after old ones and ailing family members. Presently majority of women spend more than 15 hours daily while few years back their mother spend half of this time for the same because water, fuel and fodder were easily available nearby the villages with the good cooperation from their male counterpart. Unfortunately in present time majority of the male population accomplish their ancestrally ordained work of ploughing and do nothing except this. It is also noticed that young male people were found in playing the cards or gamble.

Because of the continuous and strenuous working hours and repeated pregnancies women fall under the grip of moderate to severe mal and under nutrition and consequently they suffer from various health problems. The hypothesis of the present study are:-

1. The environmental factors decide the crop and crop production of any area the consumption pattern is found in accordance with the cropping system.
2. Consumption pattern and dietary habits decide the nutrition status of the people (women).
3. The women nutritional requirements are depend on their age, occupation, stages – general (non-lactating and non-pregnant), pregnant and lactating etc.
4. The effect of nutrient intake deficiency directly comes on the deficiency diseases and mal nutrition.
5. The under-nourished women tend to deliver low birth weight babies and have pregnancy complications.
6. The housing condition, environmental sanitation and personal hygienic sense indicate the awareness and would decide the disease pattern among the people.
7. The mal nutrition among the women determines the morbidity and mortality.
8. Through awareness campaign about the importance of personal hygiene, housing condition, environmental sanitation, modification in food habits, nutritional level and finally health status of the women in the region can be improved to some extent.

1.5 Research Design and Methodology

The main aim of the statistical sampling is to obtain, representative sampling of the rural women population as possible from each stratum so that the data collection regarding the socio-economic conditions, demographic profile, housing condition, environmental sanitation, hygiene pattern, dietary intake, food habits and nutritional status may closely reflect the situation as it exists in overall women. Random sampling procedures have been adopted to collect the authentic and relevant information.

1.5.1 Regional Division

From the Gangetic Plain in the south to a comparatively less elevated rainshadow zone of Trans Himalaya in the north, Uttarakhand Himalaya possesses a great physical diversity. For the present study the region has been divided into six latitudinal divisions Tarai, Bhabar, the Siwalik and Dun, the Lesser Himalaya, the Great Himalaya and the Trans Himalaya. Among these divisions there are number of differences concerning soil type, cropping pattern, density of population, infrastructural development, relief, climate etc. The study of 136 sample women from fourteen villages – three villages selected from Tarai, three from Bhabar, two from Dun, five from the Lesser Himalaya and last one village represents the Great Himalaya – lies close to the Great Himalaya has been completed during the specified period of Marh 1999 – February 2001. It is worth to mention that no sample village has been studied from the Trans Himalaya.

1.5.2 Selection of the Sample Women

Among the married women between the age of 15 to 59 years, ten sample except six sample women from village Bharatpur No. 1 of three categories – general, pregnant and lactating from all segments of the society have been randomly selected from the sample villages. A total 136 sample women – 39 general category, 44 pregnant and 53 lactating category women from the fourteen sample villages have been selected for the detailed study.

1.5.3 Method of Data Collection and Analysis

Data pertaining to socio-economic base, housing condition, environmental sanitation pattern, hygiene pattern, food intake etc. of the sample has been collected with the help of well structured questionnaires during door to door survey in 1999-2000. Overall information of the region has been gathered from secondary sources – statistical diaries, censuses, Survey of India Topographical Sheets, geological literature etc. Each food items taken by the women has been collected in local units and then converted into standard units in gram and milligram and finally converted into various nutrients-energy, protein, fat, carbohydrates, mineral and vitamins with the help of food composition tables and then percentage departure has been compared with the standard requirement for each group (stages) separately (Gopalan *et al.* 1993). For the calculation of Body Mass Index (BMI), height and weight have been measured at the time of survey. Body Mass Index has been calculated using the formula weight (kg)/height^2(m) and then classified into several degrees of Chronic Energy Deficiency (CED) as defined by James *et al.* (1988). The findings have been displayed in cartographic representation such as diagrams, maps etc.

1.5.4 Tools to be Used in the Collection of Data

Physical environmental study has been done with the help of Survey of India Topographical Sheets, Forest records, geological maps, literature and direct observations. Information of the overall pertaining to demography, landuse, agriculture, livestock, horticulture, amenities etc. has been gathered from the secondary sources such as statistical handbooks, census etc. Information of the sample women pertaining caste, age, literacy, occupation, workload, sanitation, hygiene, food intake habits, food consumption, behavioral tendency etc. has been collected and noted during the field work with help of questionnaires and observations. Height and weight of the sample women have been measured with the support of the measuring tape and potable weighing machine. Food items taken by the women have been measured into local units (*nali-ser, glass* etc.) and then converted into standard units of kg, grams, milligrams etc. with the help of conversion formula.

1.6 Relevance to the Present Day Problems and Needs of the Society and the Country

Despite the development in terms of infrastructural set-up and increases in food production in recent decades in general, the health status of the people and women in particular has gone bad to worse. A human being needs a wide range of nutrients to keep her/him healthy and active, most of these nutrients derive from his/her daily intake. Due to inadequate of various nutrients such as energy, protein, fat, minerals and vitamins, majority of the people suffer from under nutrition and malnutrition. Women are most affected segment of this nutritional consequences. So far as the nutritional requirements are concerned women have the additional burden of the bearing and rearing children during their reproductive periods, menstrual cycles, pregnancy and lactation, the nutritional needs of women increase significantly to meet the extra demand of these additional physiological stresses. But these aspects have been ignored in present study region. As a result of this women suffered a lot of health problems. The present investigation would be helpful to understand the causes of these consequences and would propose applicable remedies to overcome these fatal problems. The present study would also be useful for planners and policy makers of the country and region at the time when the health and nutritional problems of women are concerned. Therefore an exercise of this nature is very necessary and relevant.

1.7 The Study Area

The Himalaya constitutes one of the greatest and youngest folded mountain systems in the world rising from 200 m to more than 8000 m above sea level. The Himalaya makes the northern boundary of India extending from eastern border of Pakistan to the western border of Myanmar and having length of 2500 km and width varying from 250 to 400 km. The Himalaya encompasses an area of about five lakh km^2. From east to west it has been divided into four sections 560 km long Punjab Himalaya extends from Indus to Sutlej, 320 km Kumaun Himalaya extends from the Sutlej to the Kali (Sharda), 800 km long Nepal Himalaya lies between the Kali and the Tista and 820 km long Assam Himalaya extend from the Tista to the Myanmar (Brahmputra) or eastern most border of Arunachal Pradesh (Burrared *et al.* 1933, Pant, 1995a and 1998).

Table 1.1. Uttarakhand Himalaya: At a Glance

Particulars	Districts/Region								
	Uttarkashi	*Chamoli*	*Tehri*	*Dehradun*	*Pauri*	*Pithoragarh*	*Almora*	*Nainital*	*Uttarakhand*
Total Area (Km^2)	8016	9125	4421	3088	5440	8856	5385	6794	51125
Inahbited village (No.)	669	1516	1953	743	3237	2174	3019	1806	15117
Development Block (No.)	06	11	10	06	15	12	14	15	89
Tehsil (No.)	04	07	05	04	06	06	05	08	45
Urban Unit* (No.)	03	08	04	16	08	05	05	25	74
Population (1991)	2,39,709	4,54,871	5,80,153	10,25,679	6,82,535	5,66,408	8,36,617	15,40,174	59,26,146
Rural (%)	92.80	91.90	94.33	49.74	88.11	92.56	93.60	67.34	78.30
Urban (%)	7.20	8.91	5.67	50.26	11.89	7.44	6.40	32.66	21.70
Density (P/km^2)	30	48	130	329	123	63	153	233	115
Total Literacy**(%)	47.23	61.08	48.38	69.50	65.35	59.01	58.66	56.62	59.58
Male Lietracy (%)	68.74	82.01	72.10	77.95	82.46	79.44	79.96	67.88	75.51
Female Literacy (%)	23.51	40.37	26.41	59.26	49.44	38.37	39.60	43.19	42.58
Scheduled Caste (%)	22.78	17.49	14.20	13.40	13.52	20.45	22.02	15.80	16.70
Scheduled Tribe (%)	0.96	2.26	0.11	8.20	0.22	3.23	0.33	5.84	3.54

Source: Anon, 1991a and 1991b.

Note: 1. New districts of Udham Singh Nagar, Champawat, Bageshwar, and Rudraprayag have not been considered separately. Related information of these districts are included in their parent districts.
* Census town ** excluding below 7 years population.

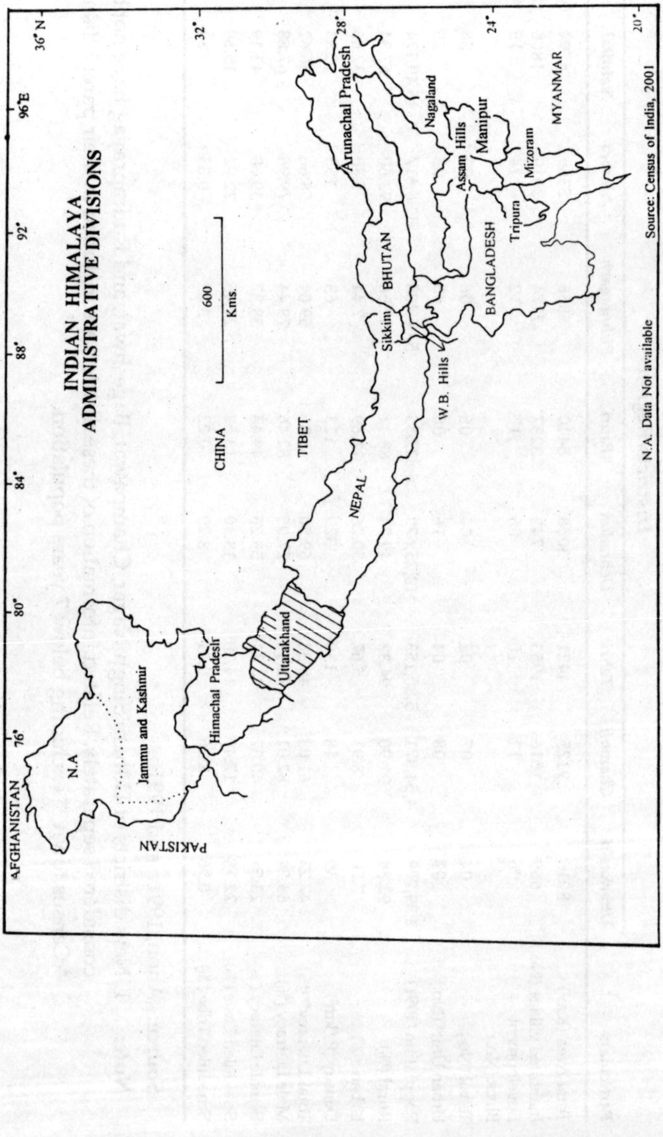

Fig. 1.1. Location of Uttarakhand in the Indian Himalaya.

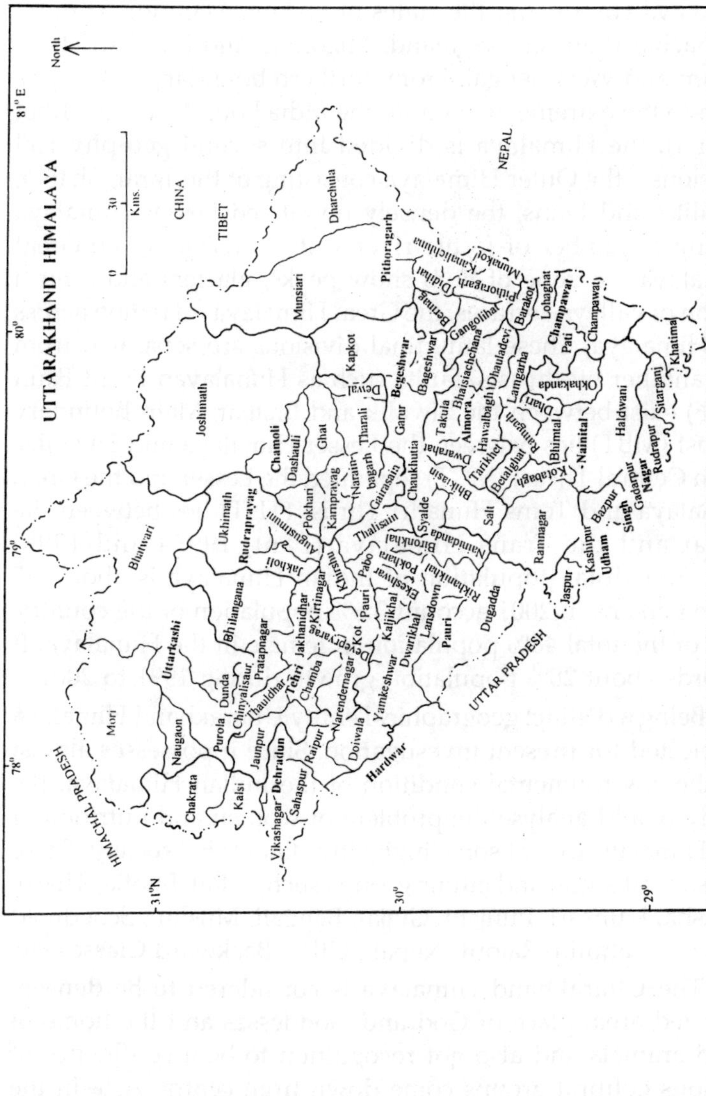

Fig. 1.2. Administartive Units of Uttarakhand Himalaya.

The Planning Commission of India (1982) has also divided the Himalaya into three broad regions – the Western Himalaya consisting of the States of Jammu & Kashmir and Himachal Pradesh, the Central Himalaya consisting of Kumaun and Garhwal divisions (Uttarakhand), and North Eastern Himalaya comprising the states of Sikkim, Manipur, Tripura, Arunachal Pradesh, Nagaland, Mizoram, and hill districts of Assam and West Bengal. From northern boundary of Gangtic Plain to the extreme north upto the India boundary with Tibet (China), the Himalaya is divided into several geo-physical divisions – the Outer Himalaya consisting of the Tarai, Bhabar, Siwaliks and Duns, the densely populated Lesser Himalaya having a number of fertile river valleys, terraces, the Great Himalaya – a zone of high snow peaks, glaciers and a birth region of valleys, terraces, the Great Himalaya – a region across the Himalaya. These latitudinal divisions are separated from one another by thrusts/faults such as Himalayan Front Fault (HFF) exist between the Siwalik and Bhabar, Main Boundary Thrust (MBT) lies between the Lesser Himalaya and Siwaliks, Main Central Thrust (MCT) separated the Lesser and the Great Himalaya and Trans Himadri Thrust (THT) lies between the Great and the Trans Himalaya (Pant, 1995a and 1998) (Fig. 3.1). Total population of Indian Himalaya is about 3.5 crore persons in 2001 account 3.6% population of the country. Out of the total 48% population in female in the Himalaya. It records about 28% population growth during 1991 to 2001.

Being a distinct geographical entity Uttarakhand Himalaya is selected for present investigation. Since it possesses almost all the environmental condition of the Indian Himalaya, the study would analyse the problem of women and nutrition of the Himalaya except some high altitudinal tribal society. These are several social and ethnic groups such as Raj, Bhotia, Tharu, Buksha, Jaunsari, Punjabi, Gujjar, Bengali, Muslim, Scheduled Castes, Brahmin, Rajput, Nepali, Other Backward Classes etc.

The Uttarakhand Himalaya is considered to be densely forested area, place of God and Goddesses and the home of wild animals and also got recognition to be a confluence of various cultural groups come down from central Asia in the north and the Gangetic Plain in the south. It extends from the Tons-feeder of Yamuna River in the west to the Kali or Sharda in the east. Its northern boundary is demarcated by Indo-Tibet water parting ridge and southern boundary corresponds almost with the southern limit of Tarai belt separating it from Saharanpur, Haridwar, Bijnor, Muradabad, Rampur, Bareilly, and Pilibhit districts (Fig. 1.2). Administratively, Uttarakhand Himalaya includes 12 districts of newly created Uttaranchal State. Historically, the region under the present study has been divided into two divisions – Kedarkhand and Manaskhand – presently Kedarkhand includes the districts of Dehradun, Uttarkashi, Tehri, Rudraprayag, Chamoli, and Pauri and Manaskhand spreads over the districts of Almora, Bageshwar, Pithoragarh, Champawat, Nainital and Udham Singh Nagar. Lying between 28°44′ and 31°25′ North latitudes and 77°45′ and 81°1′ East longitudes, it encompasses an area of 51125 Km^2 and a population of 70.35 lakh persons in 2001 (Fig. 1.2). Approximately 3074 km^2 of land form the Almora district, 2311 km^2 Bageshwar district, 3422 km^2 Nainital, 3372 km^2 Udham Singh Nagar district, 7212 km^2 Pithoragarh, 1642 km^2 Champawat, 7626 km^2 Chamoli, 3088 km^2 Dehradun, 5397 km^2 Pauri, 3796 km^2 Rudraprayag, 8016 km^2 Uttarkashi districts. Out of total population in 2001, there are 12,79,083 person in Dehradun, 12,34,548 in Udham Singh Nagar, 7,62,912 in Nainital, 6,96,851 in Pauri, 4,62,149 in Pithoragarh, 6,04,608 in Tehri, 3,69,198 in Chamoli, 2,94,179 in Uttarkashi, 2,49,453 in Bageshwar, 2,27,461 in Rudraprayag 6,30,446 in Almora and 2,24,461 person in Champawat district (Anon, 2001).

It is worth to mention that 136 sample women from 14 villages of Kumaun Himalaya (Manaskhand) were selected for detailed study. As already mention that new Uttaranchal state came in to existence on 9th November 2000 including a Hardwar additional district of Uttarakhand region. In the present study Hardwar district has not been included due to the paucity of relevant data while new districts – Udham Singh Nagar, Bageshwar, Champawat and Rudraprayag have not been considered separately. All these newly formed districts are included in their parent districts.

2

Indian Himalaya: Demographic Profile

2.1 Introduction

The Himalaya lying in Indian sub-continent constitutes one of the greatest and youngest folded mountain system in the world rising from about 300 m to more than 8000 m above sea level. It is a mountain region of majestic grandeur and high geographical significance. It acts as protector, regulator and creator of natural resources, climate and soil. The rapid increasing population, settlement and development is exhibiting environmental transformation in the form of deteriorating environment, depletion of natural resources and conditions of poverty. There has been large scale of deforestation, overgrazing and expansion of agriculture on forest and marginal lands, resulting of micro-climatic changes, loss of wild life, change in water level and river regions, soil erosion, flood and landslides, all of which brought about hardships and increasing environmental degradation in the ecologically fragile and geologically sensitive Himalayan region. Although increasing population is not solely responsible factor, while less enlightened government and non-government agencies and unawareness of the people are equally liable for this degradational process.

The Himalaya which plays a vital role not only in Indian but also in sub-continental economy is in the grip of environmental degradation. Aspects of population, which are highly correlated with it, are discussed here in this attempt with an overview of environmental profile. Figures pertaining to demographic scenario are based on census, 1991 and 2001 and overview regarding the environmental stress is based on published work.

The Himalaya makes the northern boundary of India extending from eastern border of Pakistan to the western frontiers of Myanmar and having a length of about 2500 km and width of about 160 to 400 km. Extending between 70°47′ and 97°22′ east longitudes and 21°57′ and 37°15′ north latitudes, the Himalaya encompasses in India an area of about 5,17,733 km^2 i.e. 15.75% of the country land area. Administratively the Indian Himalaya is divided into three broad regions––the Western Himalaya consisting the states of Jammu and Kashmir and Himachal Pradesh, includes illegal occupation of Pakistan and China, the Central Himalaya consisting of Uttaranchal, and the Eastern Himalaya comprising the states of Sikkim, Arunachal Pradesh, Manipur, Tripura, Mizoram, Nagaland and hill districts of Assam and West Bengal (Fig. 2.1). It is worth to mention here that the Himalayan region of West Bengal Hills consists of Darjiling district only and the Assam Hills consists of the districts of Hailakandi, Karimganj and Cachar and south eastern part of North Cachar Hills, Karbi Aonglong and north eastern part of North Cachar Hills of Assam is a part of the Meghalaya-Mikir region, i.e. eastern extension of Chhota Nagpur plateau, Cachar-Tripura plains though continuations of Barak Valley. Owing to their locational, functional, administrative and some socio-cultural contiguity and small size have been included in the Himalayan region. About 15% area of the Uttaranchal state (partially plain Dehradun, Pauri, Nainital and fully plain Hardwar and Udham Singh Nagar) is below 600 metres i.e. continuation of Indo-gengetic plain, Tarai and Bhabar.

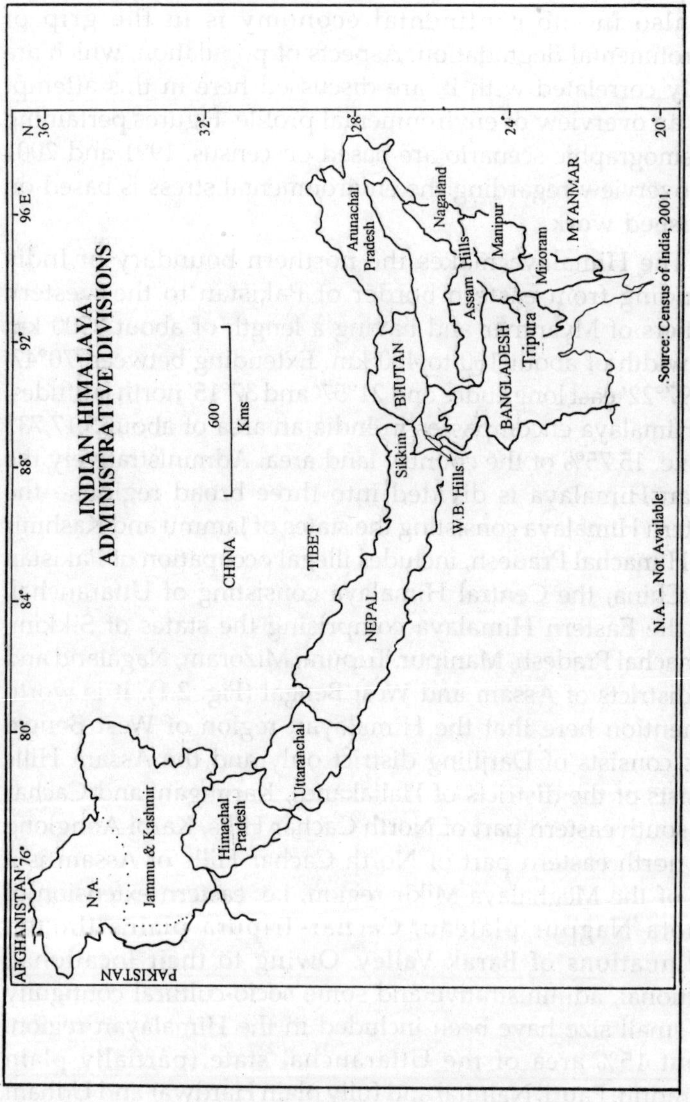

Fig. 2.1 Location of Indian Himalaya.

From the northern boundary of the alluvial plain to the extreme north upto the Indian boundary, the Himalaya is divided into several geo-tectonic divisions—the Outer Himalaya (Siwaliks, Duns, Dwars, Tarai and Bhabar), the Lesser Himalaya having a number of fertile river valleys, the Great Himalaya a zone of high snow peaks, glaciers and source of several rivers, and the Trans Himalaya a region across the Himalaya (rain shadow zone). These latitudinal divisions are separated from one another by thrusts and faults such as Himalayan Frontal Fault (H.F.F.) extending between the Siwaliks and the Bhabar, Main Boundary Thrust (M.B.T.) lying between the Siwaliks and the Lesser Himalaya, Main Central Thrust (M.C.T.) separating the Lesser and the Great Himalaya and Trans Himadri Thrust (T.H.T.) lying between the Great and the Trans Himalaya. The total population of the Indian Himalaya is 4,03,11,039 persons in 2001 accounting for about 3.92% population of the country.

2.2 Degrading Environmental Profile

With the alarming devastation caused by massive landslides, accelerating soil erosion, reducing soil productivity, drying up springs, frequent earthquakes and uncontrolled floods, the Himalaya is facing a number of environmental hazards which are manifestations of ruthless deforestation, rapid growth of population, negligence of administration and unawareness of the society on environmental issues.

The Himalayan rivers are eroding catchment areas at the mean rate of 0.1 cm per year i.e. 100 cm in 1000 year, which is five times faster than it was in recent geological past (Menard, 1963). The Ganga alone at Kolkata carries annually 411 m.t. of sediments (324 m.t. in suspended state and 83 m.t. as dissolved chemical load), implying erosion in the catchments at a rate of 549 t/km^2/yr (Abbas and Subramanian, 1984). The construction of 44000 km road in the Himalaya generates about 2640 m^3 of debris (Valdiya, 1985). About 39% of the road bed is affected by rockfall and 38% by slamping, i.e. about 24 debris chutes/km^2 (Haigh *et al.*, 1989). At the average rate of 550 m^3/km/

year the total landslide debris on Himalayan roads would be of the order of 24 m^3 annually (Valdiya, 1987). Haigh (1984) discovered 72 landslides larger than 10 m^3 and total sediment yield of 1105 m^3/km along 6 km reach of Mussoorie-Tehri road in 1978. It is well known that the whole Himalaya is dissected by various faults and thrusts. These areas are vulnerable for landslides, slumping, mass wasting etc. Similar micro studies have been conducted by the several geologists and geographers in the whole Himalaya (Ives and Messerti, 1989).

The Himalaya also suffers from overgrazing problem. For instance, this incidence in Uttaranchal Himalaya is 2.4 to 4.5 times higher than the carrying capacity of forest (Singh and Saxena, 1980). The annual depletion of forest is amounting to 3.76 million m^3 per year, i.e. at the rate of 5.8% per year (Shah, 1982). An interpretation of land imagery indicates that only 28.7% of Indian Central Himalaya is now forested and only 4.4% of the area has a forest with greater than 60% crown density (Singh *et al.,* 1984). Maximum land degradation occurs in the civil forest areas because of uncontrolled and unscientific anthropogenic activities. The degradation of forest has accelerated soil erosion tragic landslides in an unprecedented manner (Bahuguna, 1981) and floods in the adjoining plains (Reiger, 1981 and Ashish, 1983). It is estimated that out of the total net sown area of 7.32×10^5 ha, about 6.40×10^5 ha of agricultural land already suffers from severe erosion problem (Shah, 1982). The land used for agriculture is gradually being lost (Reiger, 1981). It is predicted that at the rate of 3.9 quintals per capita consumption, the carrying capacity of forest will be overreaches by 2031 AD (Shah, 1982). There is a perceptible decrease in spring discharge and seepage in more than 40% of the villages in *Guala* catchment of Kumaun Himalaya. The extent of this decrease is between 25% and 73% in the past 5 to 50 years (Valdiya and Bartarya, 1991). Evergrowing is leading to more farming and the cultivated area and the cattle population is increasing at the rate of 1.5% and 0.18% per year respectively (Shah, 1982).

The carrying capacity of the Himalaya is decreasing day by day due to the heavy pressure of both human and livestock population and consequently a large number of youths are migrating to other more developed parts of the country (Pant, 1992, 1994, 1995 and 1996c).

Majority of the rural people do not get sufficient nutrition in their diet consequently they suffered from nutrition deficiency related diseases (Pant 1994, 1996 and 1998). The largest number of epicenters is located in the Himalayan belt where the strongest seismicity is attributed to the movements along the MBT and MCT (Valdiya, 1992). The Himalaya falls under the 4th and 5th maximum intensity earthquake prone zone. The water discharge of the river Dabka in Kumaun Himalaya is decreased by 39.45% during the period of 1976-80. At this decrease continues for next 15 years, many such streams would be dry except in the monsoon seasons (Pant and Jalal, 1992). The change in micro climate is also noticed in the Himalaya. The glaciers are receding very rapidly. A number of vegetational and wild animal species are in the endangered stage.

Environmental hazards are not merely natural disasters but these are the result of increasing human activities and less visionary plannings of the development agencies.

2.3 Demographic Profile

Based on 1991 and 2001 censuses, the present study highlights the changing scenario of population structure of the Himalaya. Nepal and Bhutan could not be studied as desired due to unavailability of reliable and complete data. Basically the present study is worked out with the help of 1991 and 2001 censuses in Jammu and Kashmir, Himachal Pradesh, Uttaranchal, Sikkim, Arunachal Pradesh, Nagaland, Mizoram, Tripura, Manipur and Hills of Assam and West Bengal (see notes at the end of the chapter).

2.3.1 Distribution

The distributional pattern of the population structure differs from one place to another. These sectoral aspects are particularly determined by the environmental conditions which have both restrictive and permissive connections to human activities. Mostly the population of the Himalaya is concentrated Tarai, Bhabar, Duns, Dwars and lower valleys of the rivers, owing to their favourable environmental conditions such as conducive climate, availability of drinking water, fertile soil, well irrigational provisions and infrastructurally more developed while the mountainous parts are possessing adverse conditions and steep inclines is sparsely populated. According to the 2001 census, populations wise Jammu and Kashmir stands the largest state in the Himalaya accounts, 0.98% of the country's population. The second largest state is Uttaranchal with a population of 84,79,562 persons, which is 0.83% of the country's population. The smallest state is Sikkim with a population of 5,49,493 persons in 2001 which is 0.05% of the total population. Among other smaller state Mizoram has a population of 8,91,058 accounting for 0.09% of total population of India (Table 2.1).

Table 2.1. Country's Population in the Himalaya

S. No.	*State/Region*	*Percentage of Country's Population*		
		1981	*1991*	*2001*
1.	Jammu and Kashmir	0.88	0.92	0.98
2.	Himachal Pradesh	0.63	0.61	0.68
3.	Uttaranchal	0.85	0.84	0.83
4.	Sikkim	0.05	0.05	0.05
5.	Arunachal Pradesh	0.09	0.10	0.11
6.	Nagaland	0.11	0.14	0.19
7.	Manipur	0.21	0.22	0.23
8.	Mizoram	0.07	0.08	0.09
9.	Tripura	0.30	0.33	0.31
10.	Assam Hills	N.A.	0.40	0.39
11.	West Bengal Hills	0.15	0.16	0.16

Source: Anon, 1991 (a), (b) and 2001. (Vide Note given in the end).
N.A.: Not available.

Table 2.1 shows the population distribution of 1981, 1991, and 2001, which shows almost similar pattern. The population of Jammu and Kashmir were respectively 0.88% and 0.92%, of Uttaranchal 0.85% and 0.84% and that of Himachal Pradesh were 0.63% and 0.61% of the total population in 1981 and 1991 where too Sikkim was smallest populated state in both the censuses with 0.05% of the total country population and Mizoram stood second having respectively 0.07% and 0.08% in 1981 and 1991 of India's population (Table 2.1 and Fig. 2.2).

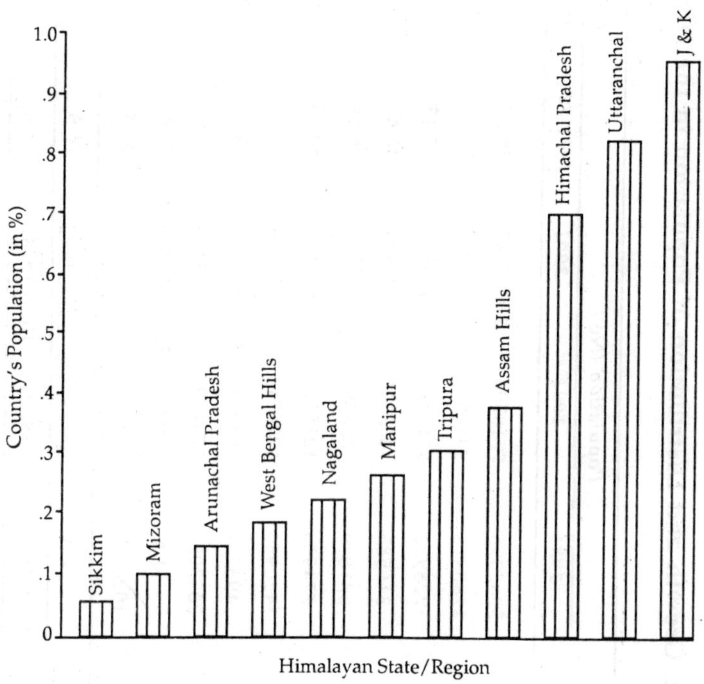

Fig. 2.2. Country's Population in the Himalayan State/Regions, 2001.

2.3.2 Growth and Density

The Indian Himalaya has registered 24.75% growth during the 1991 to 2001 which is higher than the country's average (21.34%). Among the Himalayan states/regions, Nagaland

Table 2.2. Growth and Distribution of Population in the Himalaya

S.No.	State/Region	Population (No.)			Growth (%)		
		1981	*1991*	*2001*	*1971-81*	*1981-91*	*1991-01*
1.	Jammu & Kashmir	5987398	7718700	10069917	29.59	30.34	29.04
2.	Himachal Pradesh	4280818	5111079	6077248	23.71	20.79	17.53
3.	Uttaranchal	5725972	7113483	8479562	27.45	24.23	19.20
4.	Sikkim	316585	405505	540493	N.A.	28.47	32.98
5.	Arunachal Pradesh	631839	858392	1091117	35.15	36.83	26.21
6.	Nagaland	774930	1215573	1988636	50.05	56.08	64.41
7.	Manipur	1420953	1826714	2388634	32.46	29.29	30.02
8.	Mizoram	493757	686217	891058	53.16	39.70	29.18
9.	Tripura	2053058	2744827	3191168	31.91	34.30	15.74
10.	Assam Hills	N.A.	3294770	3987306	N.A.	N.A.	21.02
11.	West Bengal Hills	1024269	1335618	1605900	N.A.	26.91	23.54
Himalaya		N.A.	32310878	40311039	N.A.	N.A.	24.75
India		6813329097	846387888	1027015247	N.A.	23.86	21.34

Source: Anon, 1991 (a), (b) and 2001.

registered maximum 64.41% growth during the decade of 1991 to 2001 which is far above the national average. Barring Manipur, Nagaland and Sikkim, decadal growth has declined in all the states/regions of the Himalaya. In case of Manipur, Nagaland and Sikkim, it has gone up respectively from 29.29%, 56.08% and 28.47% in the previous decade to 30.02%, 64.41% and 32.98% in the current decade (Table 2.2 and Fig. 2.3).

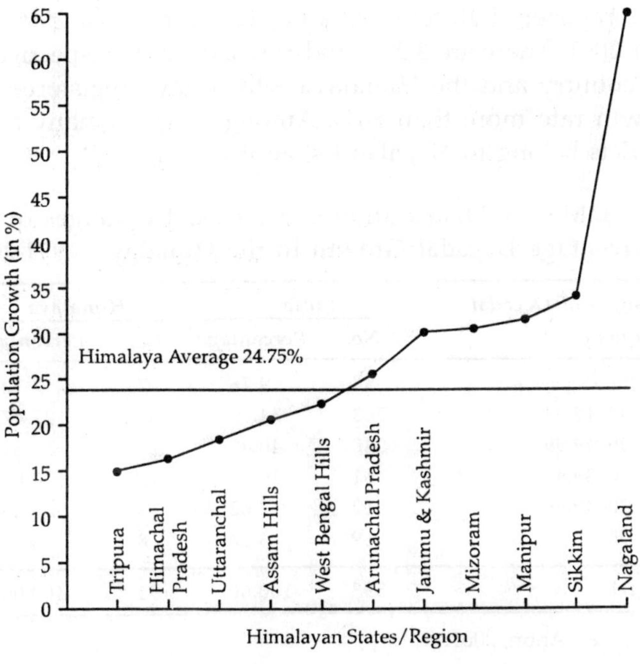

Fig. 2.3. Decadal Growth of Population in the Himalaya 1991–2001.

The main cause of this growth in these three states in immigration from the less developed areas, it may be national or international. In the rest of North Eastern states like Arunachal Pradesh, Tripura, Mizoram, Assam and West Bengal Hills, the growth is registered respectively 26.21, 15.74, 29.18, 21.02 and 23.54% which is declined from the previous decades.

The growth of population in Himalayan states/regions, only Himachal, Uttaranchal and Assam Hills, has shown less growth than the national average (Table 2.2 and Fig. 2.4).

Table 2.3 gives the distribution of the districts in each state/region of Himalaya and India by the ranges of percentage decadal growth during 1991-2001. Out of the total 7.7% districts of the Himalaya and 9.78% districts of India have registered decadal growth rate less than 10%. Maximum 74.70% districts of India and 59.34% districts of the Himalaya have registered 10 to 29.99% growth during the decade of 1991-2001. There are 3.20% and 8.79% districts respectively in the country and the Himalaya which have registered high growth rate more than 50%. Among them as many as five districts belong to Nagaland state itself (Fig. 2.5).

Table 2.3. Distribution of Districts by Ranges of Percentage Decadal Growth in the Himalaya, 1991-2001

Ranges of Decadal Growth (%)	*India*		*Himalaya*	
	No.	*Percentage*	*No.*	*Percentage*
<10.00	58	9.78	7	7.70
10.00–19.99	203	34.23	25	27.47
20.00–29.99	240	40.47	29	31.87
30.00–39.99	61	10.30	19	20.88
40.00–49.99	12	2.02	3	3.29
50.00+	19	3.20	8	8.79
Total	593	100.00	91	100.00

Source: Anon, 2001.

Density is the number of persons per km^2. For Himalaya it now works out to 78 persons/km^2 as against 62 persons/km^2 at 1991 census. This means that the pressure in the Himalaya has increased by 16 person/km^2 during the decade. The population density in the Himalaya is far less than the country average because of the rugged topography and adverse climatic conditions. Maximum area is not suitable for human habitation in the Himalaya.

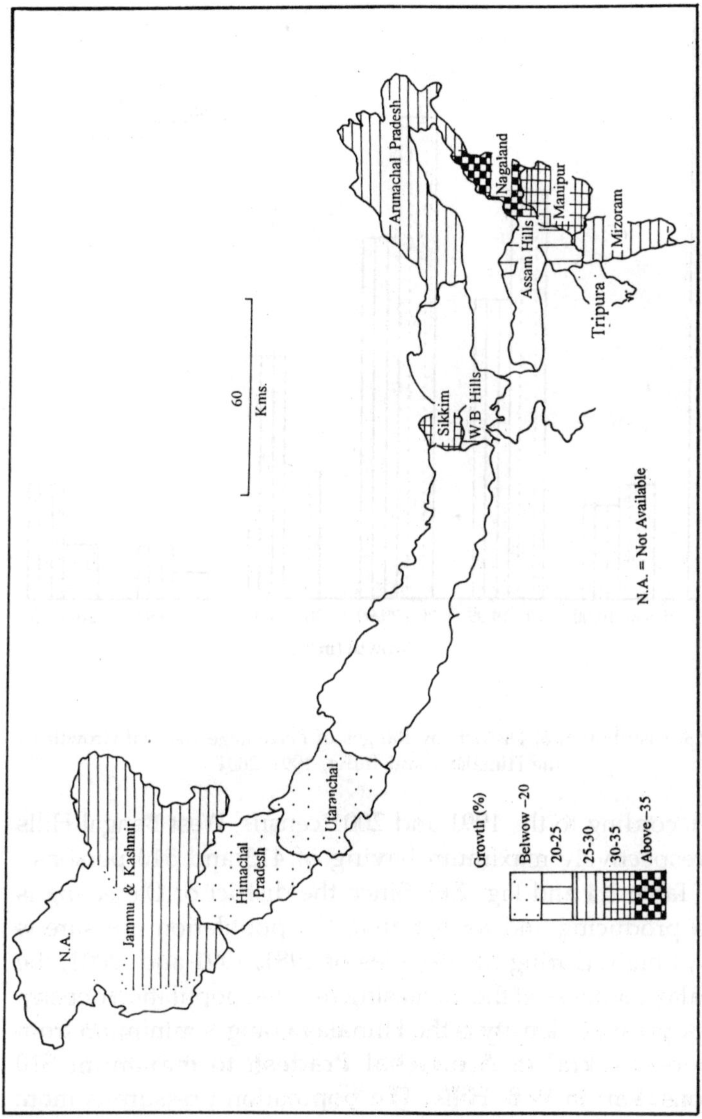

Fig. 2.4. Decadal Growth of Population in the Himalaya, 1991-2001.

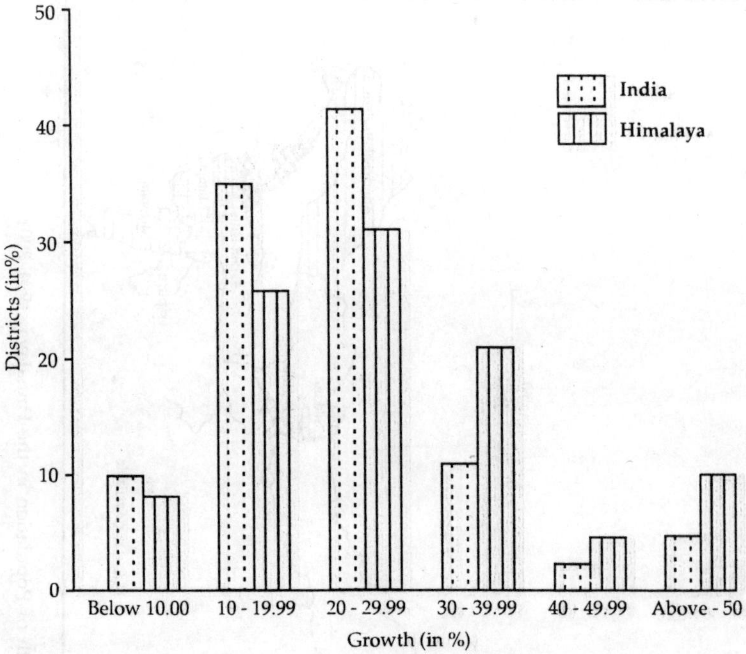

Fig. 2.5. Distribution of Districts by Ranges of Percentage Decadal Growth in the Himalaya and India, 1991–2001.

According to the 1991 and 2001 census, West Bengal Hills has respectively maximum having of 413 and 510 persons/ km² (Table 2.4 and Fig. 2.6). Since the district of Darjeeling is a Tea producing and tourist area, the population pressure is always high. During the decades of 1981, 1991 and 2001, the Himalaya witnessed the increasing trend in population density. The population density is the Himalaya ranges minimum from 13 persons/km² in Arunachal Pradesh to maximum 510 persons/km² in W.B. Hills. The population pressure is more than expected in Tripura (304 persons/km²), Hills of Assam (179) and Uttaranchal (159). In the remaining states, Himachal

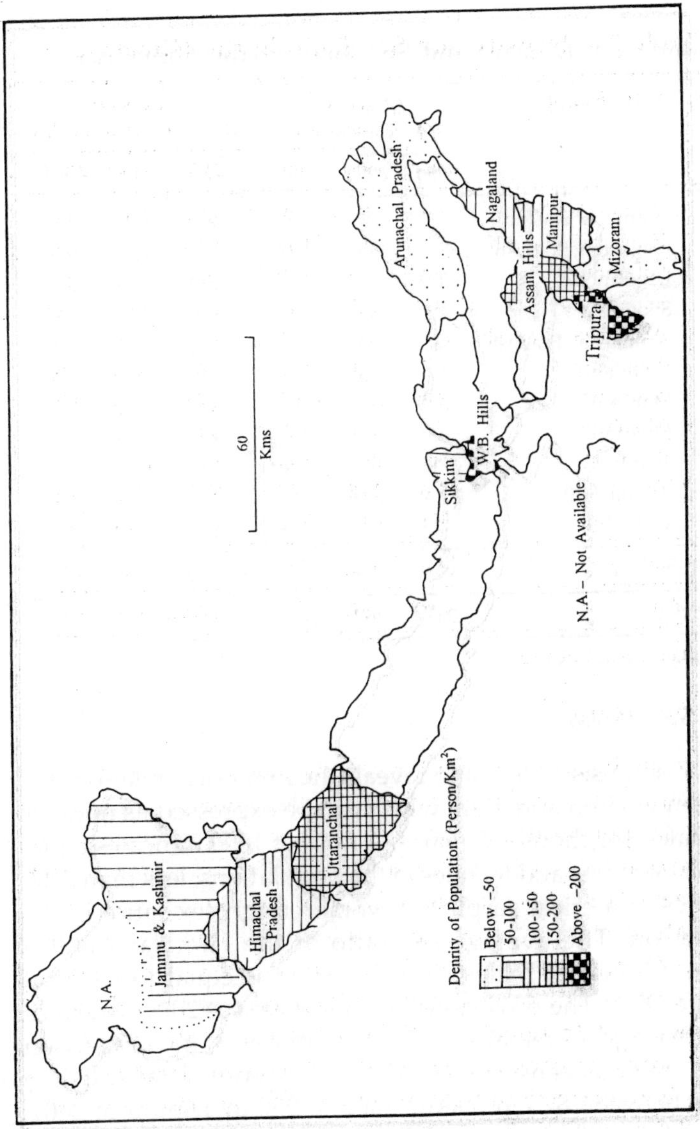

Fig. 2.6. Density of Population (Persons/Km^2) in the Himalaya, 2001.

Pradesh has density of 109 persons/km^2, Jammu and Kashmir (99) and Mizoram (42) (Table 2.4).

Table 2.4. Density and Sex Ratio in the Himalaya

S. No.	State/Region	Density (persons/km^2)			Sex Ratio (females/1000 males)		
		1981	1991	2001	1981	1991	2001
1.	Jammu & Kashmir	59	77	99	892	896	900
2.	Himachal Pradesh	77	93	109	973	976	970
3.	Uttaranchal	109	133	159	920	936	964
4.	Sikkim	45	57	76	835	878	875
5.	Arunachal Pradesh	8	10	13	862	859	901
6.	Nagaland	47	73	120	867	886	909
7.	Manipur	64	82	107	971	958	978
8.	Mizoram	23	33	42	919	921	938
9.	Tripura	196	263	304	946	945	950
10.	Assam Hills	N.A.	148	179	N.A.	930	935
11.	W.B. Hills	325	413	510	888	914	943
	Himalaya	N.A.	62	78	N.A.	918	933
	India	216	267	327	934	927	933

Source: As in table 2.1.

2.3.3 Sex Ratio

The analysis of sex ratio reveals the numerical relationship between women and men, which can be expressed as number of females per thousand males. A ratio of 1000 indicates equal balance of males and females in the populations, less than 1000 indicates numerical surplus of women (high sex ratio) in the population. The average sex ratio of the Himalaya is 933 females/thousand males in 2001, which is equal to national average (933). The provisional results of census 2001, indicates an increase of 15 females in the sex ratio (933) in comparison to the previous census (918) in the Himalaya. Total sex ratio ranges between 875 in Sikkim state to 950 in Tripura in 2001. Table 2.4 reveals that out of the total 11 states/regions in the Himalaya, 9 states/regions have shown improvement in sex ratio in comparison to previous censuses.

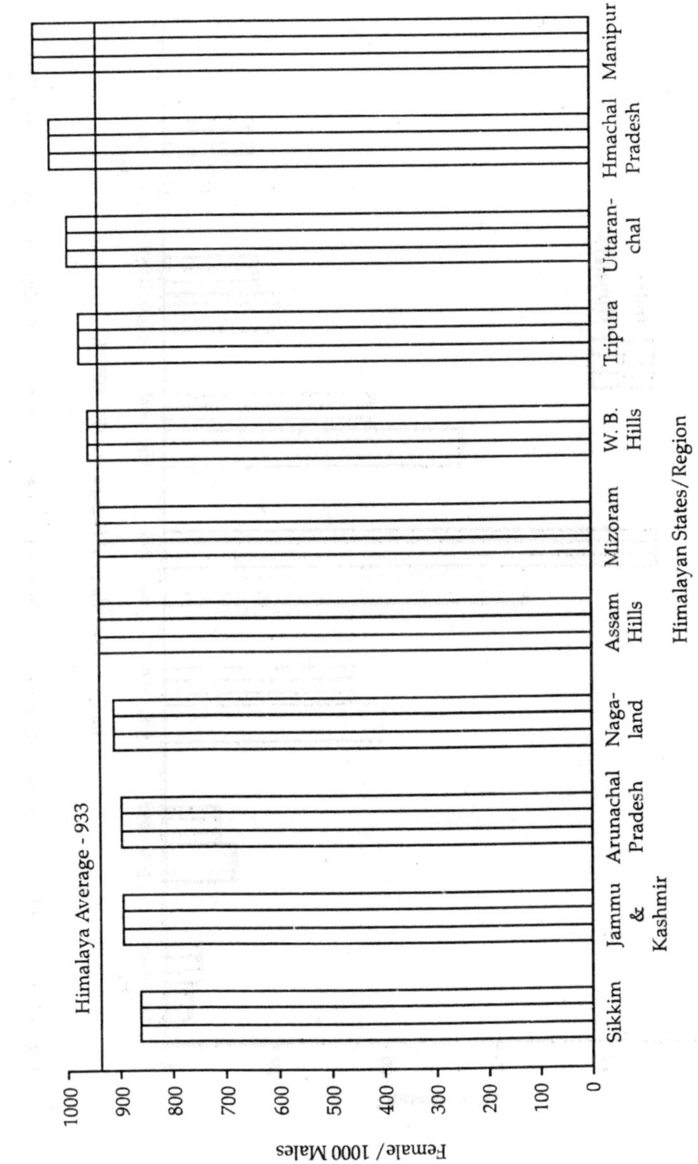

Fig. 2.7. Sex Ratio in Himalaya, 2001.

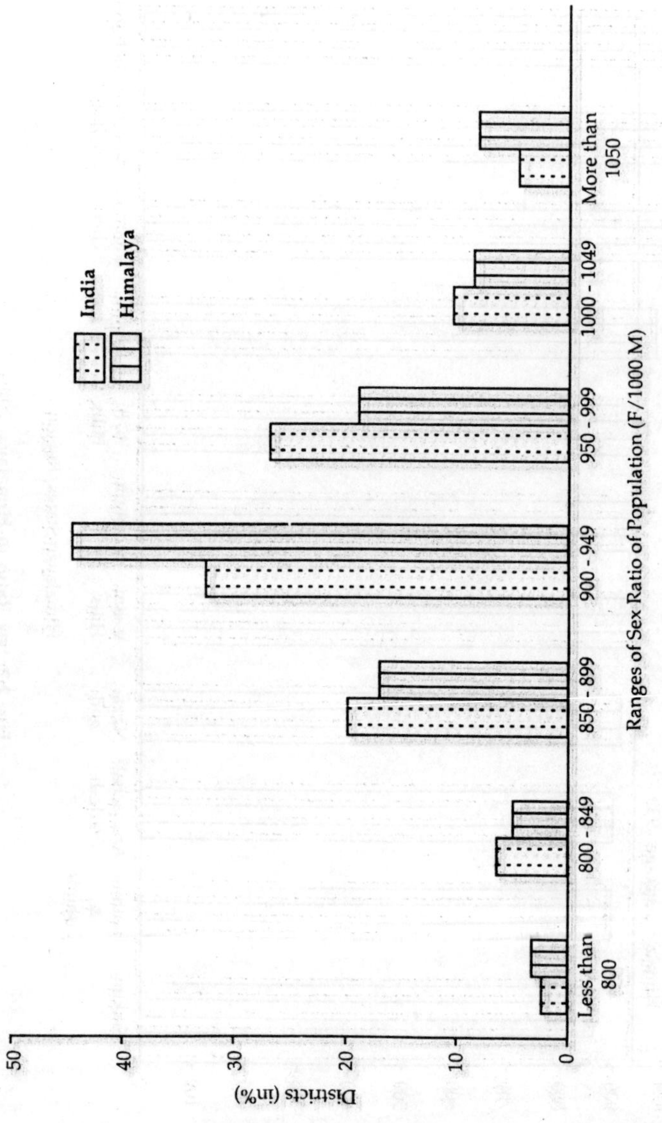

Fig. 2.8. Distribution of Districts by Ranges of Sex Ratio of Population in the Himalaya and India, 2001.

Another table 2.5, presents the distribution of districts in the ranges of sex ratio of the population of the national and Himalayan level. It is evident in this table that 26.98% of the total districts of India have sex ratio of below 900 for the total population. Similarly 23.08% of the total Himalayan districts have low sex ratio i.e. below 900 females 1000 males. It is seen that 31.15% districts at national and 14.28% at Himalaya have recorded high sex ratio (Table 2.5). The largest number of such districts in Himalaya is from Uttaranchal (8) followed by Himachal (3) while Manipur have two districts in this category. It is noteworthy that those districts having more urban population have recorded low sex ratio due to the male immigration in these districts from the less developed districts while the rural dominates districts have recorded high sex ratio due to out migration of men from the village to more developed places in search of employment and better facilities.

Table 2.5. Distribution of Districts by Ranges of Sex Ratio of Population in the Himalaya, 2001

Ranges of sex ratio (F/1000M)	*India*		*Himalaya*	
	No.	*Percentage*	*No.*	*Percentage*
Less than 800	8	1.35	2	2.20
800–849	34	5.73	4	4.40
850–899	118	19.90	15	16.48
900–949	194	32.72	40	43.96
950–999	161	27.15	17	18.68
1000–1049	58	9.78	7	7.69
1050+	20	3.37	6	6.59
Total	593	100.00	91	100.00

Source: Anon, 2001.

2.?.4 Literacy

Literacy is one of the important social aspects on which information is obtained of every individual in census. For the purpose of census 1991 and 2001 a person aged seven and above, who can both read and write with understanding any

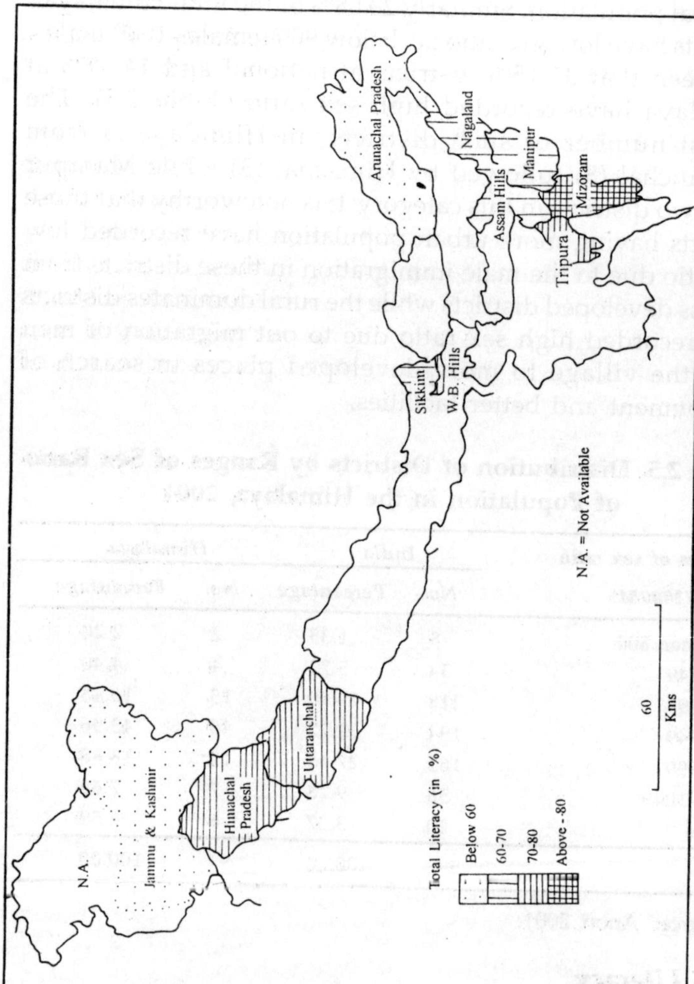

Fig. 2.9. Literacy (Persons) in the Himalaya 2001.

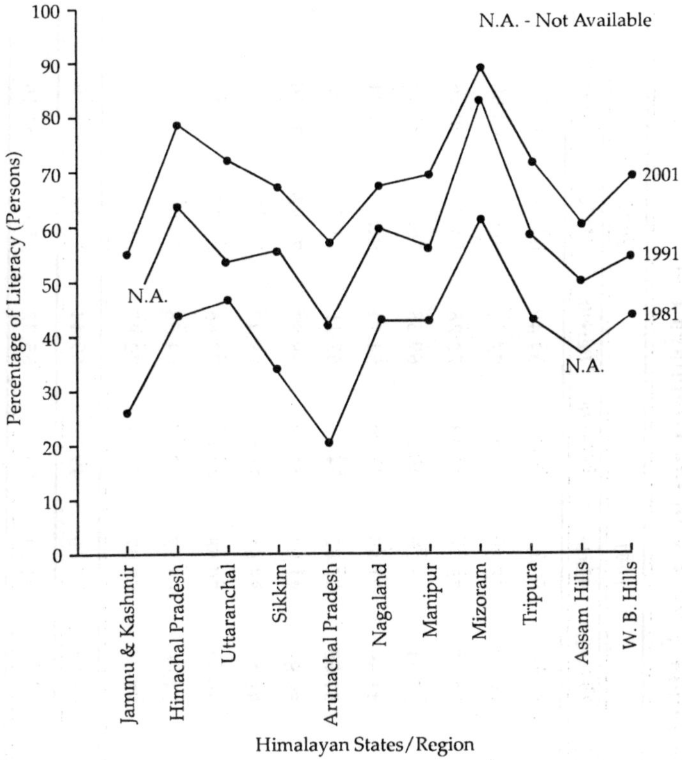

Fig 2.10. Percentage of Literacy (Persons) in the Himalaya, 1981 to 2001.

language is treated as literate. Table 2.6 shows the literacy rates for the year, 1981, 1991, and 2001. Like India, the whole Himalayan region has had an expected progress in the literacy aspect during 1981 to 1991 and 1991 to 2001. Maximum literacy is in Mizoram (88.49%) where 90.69% males and 86.13% females are literates which is quite higher than the national and Himalayan averages. It is due to the educational programmes launched by the missionaries from the earlier days of independence. Out of the total states/regions in the

Table 2.6. Literacy by Sex in the Himalaya (%)

S.No.	State/Region	1981	1991			2001		
		Person	Person	Male	Female	Person	Male	Female
1.	Jammu & Kashmir	26.66	N.A.	N.A.	N.A.	54.46	65.75	41.82
2.	Himachal Pradesh	42.47	63.86	75.36	52.13	77.13	86.02	68.08
3.	Uttaranchal	46.06	57.75	72.79	41.63	72.28	84.01	60.26
4.	Sikkim	34.05	56.94	65.70	46.76	69.68	76.73	61.46
5.	Arunachal Pradesh	20.78	41.59	51.45	29.69	54.74	64.07	44.24
6.	Nagaland	42.57	61.65	67.62	54.75	67.11	71.77	61.92
7.	Manipur	41.36	59.89	71.63	47.60	68.87	77.87	59.70
8.	Mizoram	59.88	82.27	85.61	78.60	88.49	90.69	86.13
9.	Tripura	42.12	60.44	70.58	49.65	73.66	81.47	65.41
10.	Assam Hills	N.A.	54.06	63.77	43.25	64.58	70.85	55.73
11.	West Bengal Hills	42.47	57.95	67.07	47.84	72.87	81.28	63.92
	Himalaya	N.A.	59.64	69.16	49.19	69.44	77.32	60.79
	India	43.57	52.21	64.13	39.29	65.37	75.85	54.16

Source: Anon, 1991 (a), (b) & 2001.

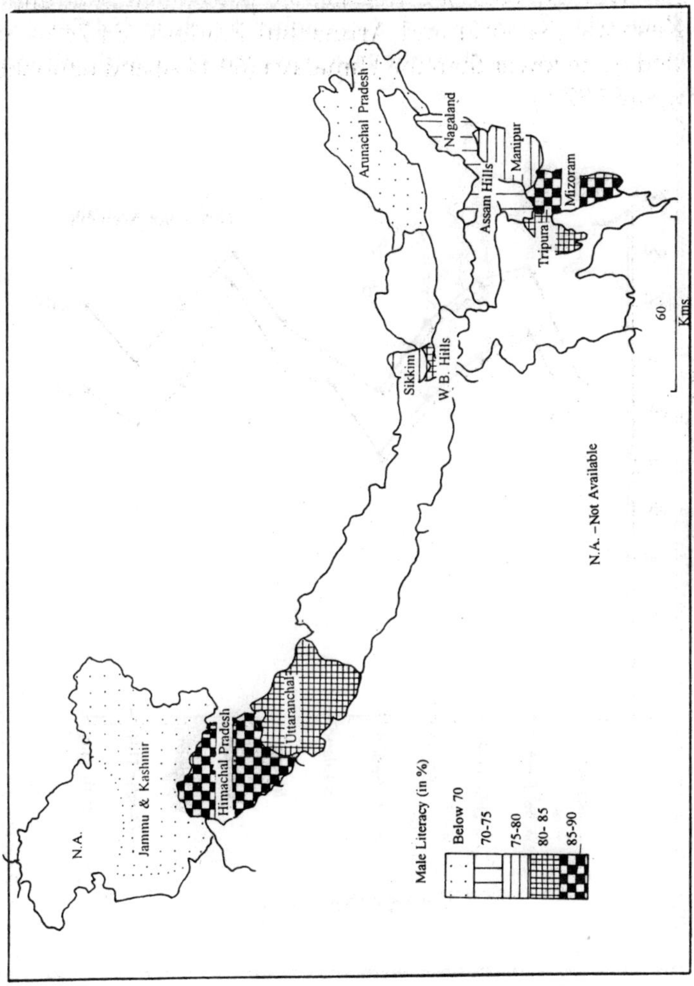

Fig. 2.11. Literacy Rate (Male) in the Himalaya 2001.

Himalaya eight states/regions-Himachal Pradesh (77.13%), Uttaranchal (72.28%), Manipur (68.87%), Nagaland (67.11%), Sikkim (69.68%), Tripura (73.66%), Mizoram (88.49%) and West Bengal Hills (72.87%) have registered higher literacy than the national average (65.37%). The literacy percentage in Jammu and Kashmir (54.46%) and Arunachal Pradesh (54.74%) is recorded quite lower than the Himalaya (69.44%) and national average (65.37%).

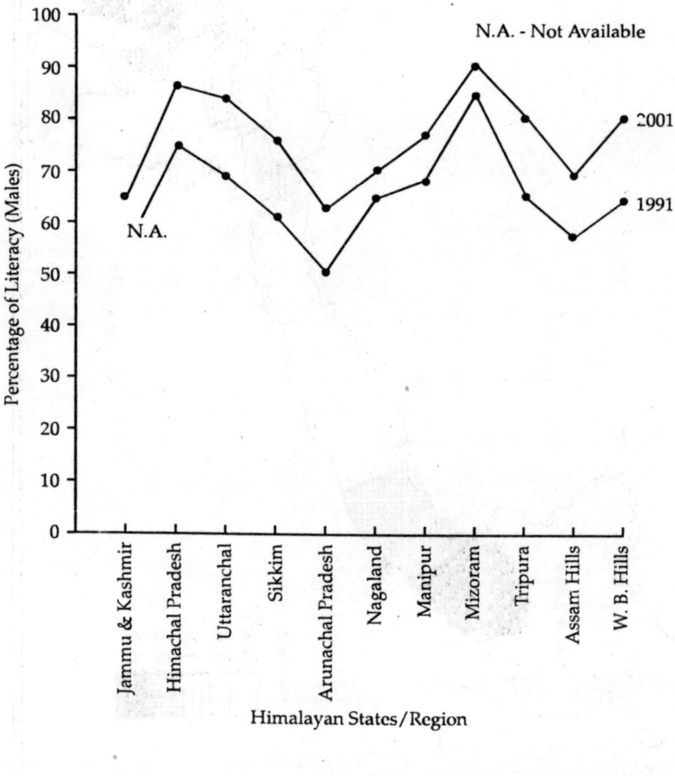

Fig. 2.12. Percentage of Literacy (Males) in the Himalaya, 1991 & 2001.

The highest proportion of male literates has been observed in Mizoram (90.69%) followed by Himachal Pradesh (86.02%).

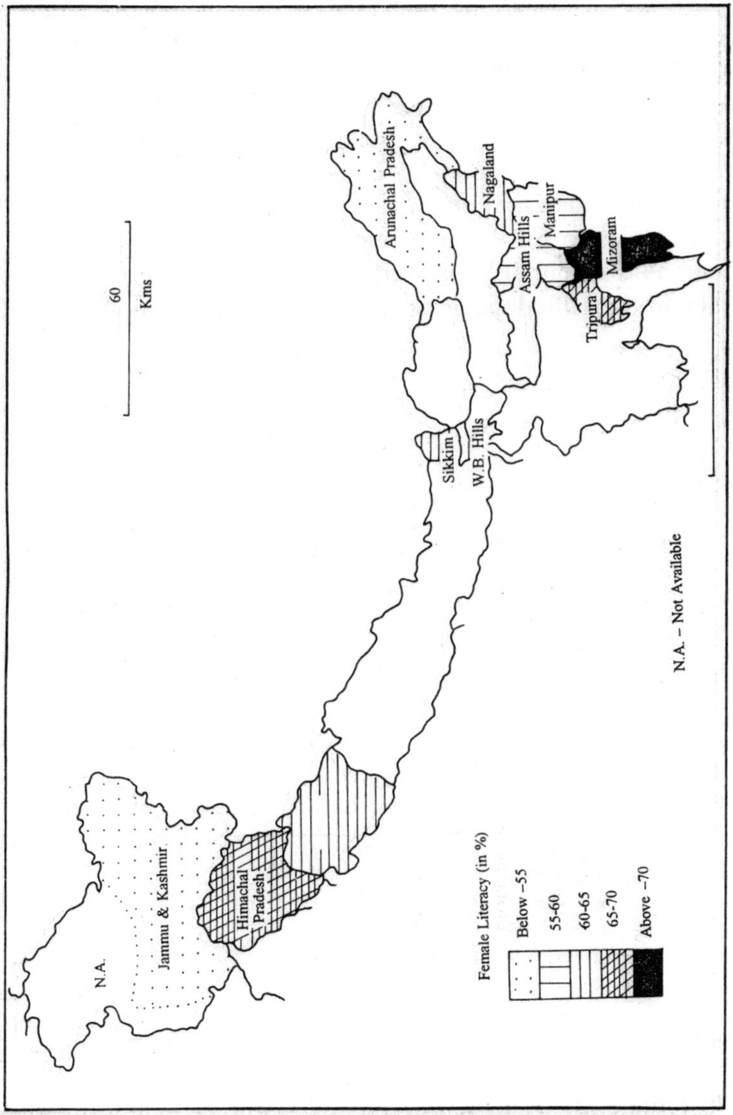

Fig. 2.13. Literacy Rate (Female) in the Himalaya, 2001

Other three states/regions with more than 80% male literacy are Uttaranchal (84.01%), Tripura (81.47%) and West Bengal Hills (81.28%). Remaining units are lying between the range of 64 to 80%. In respect of male literacy out of total seven states/regions lying above the national average (75.85%). On an average in Himalaya, the female literacy at the 1991 census was very low (49.19%). The same has now gone up to 60.79%. In fact, the improvement in female literacy has been faster (11.6% points) than that of males (8.16% points) which is quite less growth than the nation (persons 13.16, males 11.72 and females 14.8% points). This shows that momentum of female literacy in the Himalaya as well as in the whole nation.

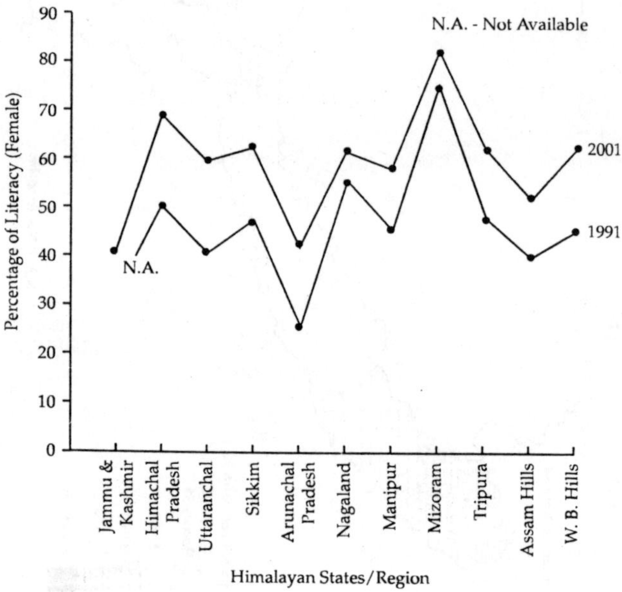

Fig 2.14. Percentage of Literacy (Female) in the Himalaya 1991 & 2001.

In female Mizoram with 86.13% literate leads among all states/regions in the Himalaya followed by Himachal (68.08%) and Tripura (65.14%). Jammu and Kashmir state has the least proportion of female literates (41.82%) followed by Arunachal Pradesh (44.2%) and Assam Hills (55.73%). Female literacy is one of the important indicators of social development.

Tables 2.7 to 2.9 give the distribution of districts in different ranges of literacy rates for persons, males and females at the national level and the Himalaya. The 4.4% districts in the country and 1.11% of Jammu and Kashmir in the Himalaya having literacy rates of below 40%. It is observed that out of total districts of the country and the Himalaya, respectively, 35.7% and 46.67% districts have registered more than 70% literacy rates. The Himalayan states/regions in which no district has been found with literacy rate below 60% are Himachal Pradesh, Uttaranchal and West Bengal Hills. The 9.98% and 14.44% districts respectively in the country and the Himalaya with literacy rate of 80% and above. These are mainly concentrated in Himachal Pradesh (3) and Mizoram (7) in the Himalaya. About 2.20% and 4.44% districts respectively in the country and the Himalaya have reported literacy rate of 90% and above. Four of these districts located in the Mizoram state of Himalaya.

Table 2.7. Distribution of Districts by Ranges of Literacy Rates (Persons) in the Himalaya, 2001

Ranges of Literacy Rate (%)	*India*		*Himalaya*	
	No.	*%*	*No.*	*%*
30.0 – 39.9	26	4.40	1	1.11
40.0 – 49.9	55	9.31	11	12.22
50.0 – 59.9	127	21.49	17	18.90
60.0 – 69.9	172	29.10	19	21.11
70.0 – 79.9	152	25.72	29	32.22
80.0 – 89.9	46	7.78	9	10.00
90.0 +	13	2.20	4	4.44
Total	591	100.00	90	100.00

Source: Anon, 2001.

There are 3.38% and 1.11% districts respectively in the country and in the Himalaya with male literacy rate below

50%. Among these one district falls in the Himalaya (Nagaland). The 70.2% districts of the country and 66.67% districts of the Himalaya have reported male literacy of 70% and above (Table 2.8).

Table 2.8. Distribution of Districts by Ranges of Literacy Rates (Male) in the Himalaya, 2001

Ranges of Literacy Rate (%)	*India*		*Himalaya*	
	No.	*%*	*No.*	*%*
30.0 – 39.9	01	0.17	–	–
40.0 – 49.9	19	3.21	01	1.11
50.0 – 59.9	46	7.78	13	14.44
60.0 – 69.9	110	18.61	16	17.78
70.0 – 79.9	190	32.15	19	21.11
80.0 – 89.9	195	33.00	32	35.56
90.0 +	30	5.08	9	10.00
Total	591	100.00	90	100.00

Source: Anon, 2001.

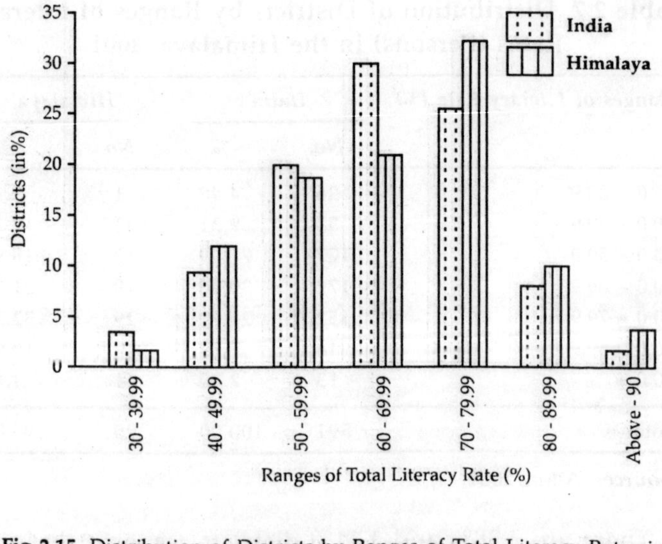

Fig 2.15. Distribution of Districts by Ranges of Total Literacy Rates in Himalaya & India, 2001.

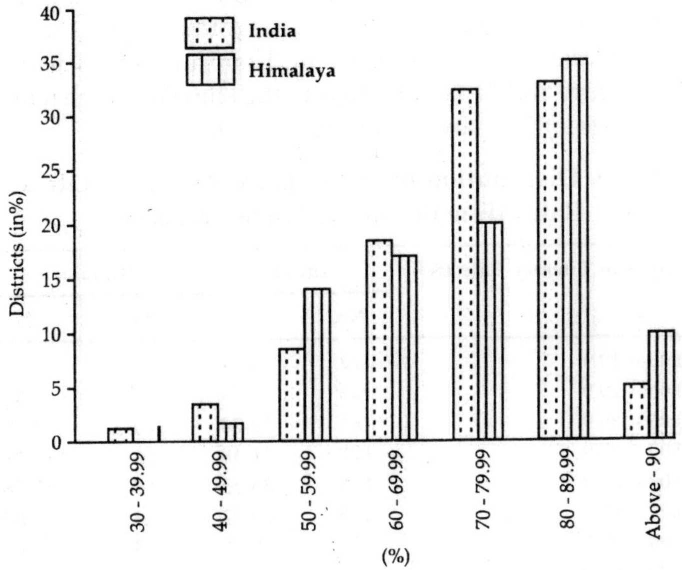

Fig. 2.16. Distribution of Districts by Ranges of Male Literacy Rates in Himalaya & India, 2001.

Table 2.8 reveals that there are 5.08% and 10% districts of the country and Himalaya with male literacy rate of 90% and above. In the Himalaya they are scattered in Himachal Pradesh (one district), Uttaranchal (4 districts) and Mizoram (4 districts).

Table 2.9 gives distribution of districts by the different ranges of female literacy rate. The 7.62% and 5.56% districts respectively in the country and in the Himalaya where the female literacy rates are still below thirty percent. Among these three districts of Jammu and Kashmir and two districts of Arunachal Pradesh located in the Himalaya. About 42.81% districts of the country and 34.44% districts of the Himalaya have registered female literacy rate below 50 percent. Out of the total 31 districts of Himalaya in this category are 11 districts located in Jammu and Kashmir out of 14 districts, in Arunachal

Pradesh 10 districts out of 13, in Assam hills one districts out of 5 districts, in Uttaranchal 2 districts out of 13, in Nagaland 2 districts out of 8, in Manipur 3 districts out of 9, and 1 district out of 8 districts located in Mizoram. There are 13.87% districts in the country and 21.11% districts in the Himalaya with female literacy rate of 70% and above (Table 2.9).

Table 2.9. Distribution of Districts by Ranges of Literacy Rates (Female) in the Himalaya, 2001

Ranges of Literacy Rate (%)	*India*		*Himalaya*	
	No.	*%*	*No.*	*%*
10.00 – 19.9	2	0.34	–	–
20.00 – 29.9	43	7.28	5	5.56
30.00 – 39.9	81	13.70	10	11.11
40.00 – 49.9	127	21.49	16	17.78
50.00 – 59.9	138	23.35	16	17.78
60.00 – 69.9	118	19.97	24	26.67
70.00 – 79.9	59	9.98	13	14.44
80.00 – 89.9	16	2.71	4	4.44
90.9 +	7	1.18	2	2.22
Total	591	100.00	90	100.00

Source: Anon, 2001.

In the Himalaya, Mizoram, Himachal Pradesh, Uttaranchal, Nagaland, Manipur and Tripura have 7, 5, 2, 1 and 1 districts respectively with female literacy rate of 70% and above. Only 1.18% of the country and 2.22% districts of the Himalaya (Mizoram) have reported female literacy rate of ninety per cent and above (Table 2.9). Traditionally, there has been some bias against female education in the Indian society and until very recently education was not usually considered important for females. The spread of modernization, urbanization and westernization associated with the nation of egalitarianism have contributed to reduction of disparity between the male and female literacy rates. However, regional disparities still exist. There is a high correlation between the male and female literacy rates. The districts with lower male literacy rate also tend to have lower female literacy rates. Generally it is also observed that districts with higher literacy rates have lower male-female disparity in literacy rates.

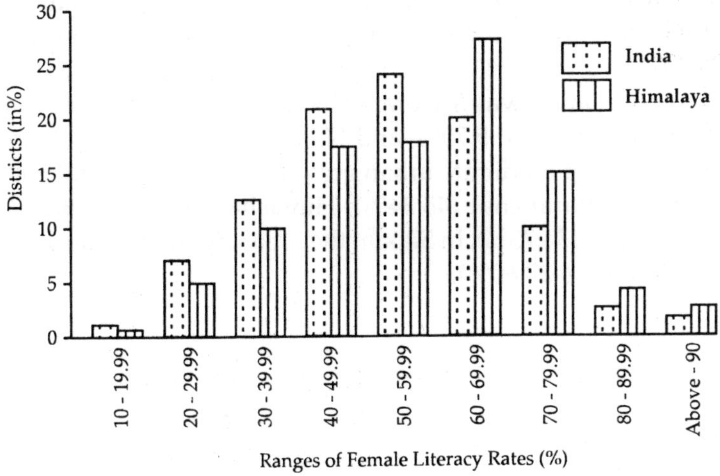

Fig. 2.17. Distribution of District by Ranges of Female Literacy Rates in Himalaya and India, 2001.

2.3.5 Urbanisation

Urban population figures for 2001 census are yet not published/available. Therefore the analysis is based on data available for census 1991. Most of the Himalayan states/regions are witnessing a slow change in the ratio of rural urban population. The Himalayan region has mostly rural population, but steadily the developing towns are attracting large proportion of this rural population. Due to facilities of tourism, trade and services in those small towns, immigration towards urban centers has considerable increased. Among Himalayan states, the maximum urban population in Mizoram where 46.2% of total population was urban. There were six towns in eight districts of Mizoram followed by West Bengal Hills (30.71%) and Manipur (27.69%) which had more than national average (25.72%) (Table 2.10). On the contrary, there were some rural population dominated regions too, the important being Himachal Pradesh, Sikkim, Assam Hills where the percentage of rural population was above 90%. Together all the states of the Himalaya only 19.91% population was urban which was quite lower than that of the national average (25.72%). During 1981-1991, the states having high growth in urban population was Mizoram (160.27%), Arunachal Pradesh (152.98%), Tripura (85.75%) and Nagaland (74.74%), while the regions having moderate urban growth were West Bengal Hills (45.38%), Uttaranchal (45.34%), Himachal Pradesh (36.46%) and Manipur (34.73%). In Sikkim the urban population declined considerably (-27.60%).

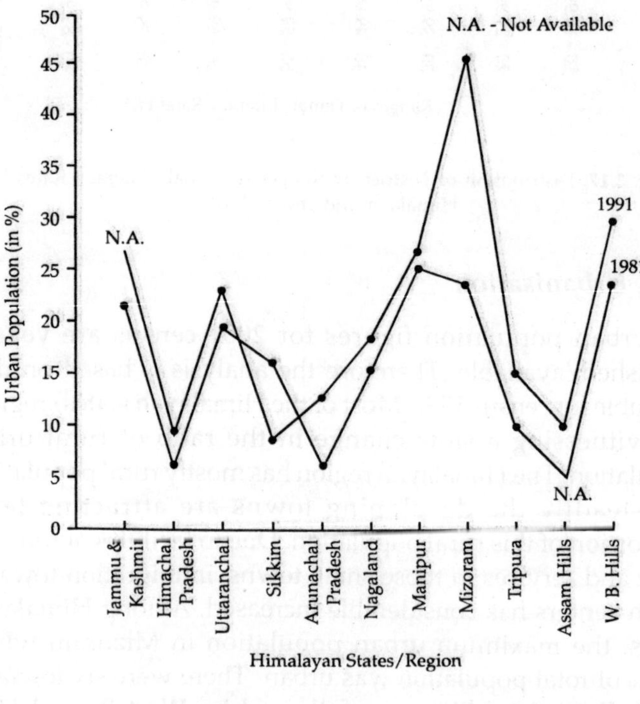

Fig. 2.18. Urban Population in the Himalaya.

Table 2.10. Rural-Urban Population in the Himalaya (%)

S.No.	*State/Region*	*1981*		*1991*	
		Rural	*Urban*	*Rural*	*Urban*
1.	Jammu & Kashmir	78.95	21.05	N.A.	N.A.
2.	Himachal Pradesh	92.38	7.62	91.30	8.70
3.	Uttaranchal	79.70	20.30	76.90	23.10
4.	Sikkim	83.85	16.15	90.88	9.12
5.	Arunachal Pradesh	93.44	6.56	87.79	12.21
6.	Nagaland	84.48	15.52	82.72	17.28
7.	Manipur	73.57	26.43	72.31	27.69
8.	Mizoram	75.33	24.67	53.08	46.20
9.	Tripura	89.01	10.99	84.74	15.26
10.	Assam Hills	N.A	N.A	90.36	9.64
11.	West Bengal Hills	72.45	27.55	69.29	30.71
	Himalaya*	82.32	17.68	80.01	19.91
	India*	76.66	23.34	74.28	25.72

Source: Anon, 1991(b). Data for 2001 are yet not published.

* Excludes Jammu and Kashmir

The study concludes that for the last many decades the Himalaya endures several environmental problems including soil erosion, deforestation, overgrazing, landslides, floods, siltation, decreasing soil fertility, drying of springs, increasing slums, health hazards etc. It can be suggested that all development efforts for the region should be made according to demographic traits and needs, and keeping in mind the carrying capacity of the resources and ecologically fragile and geologically sensitive Himalayan environment. A separate population policy should be framed for the Himalaya. Any approach adopted for planning in this region must be consider the aspects of man and his environment.

There is an urgent need to improve the education status of the people particularly of females, which is too low in the Himalayan states. More employment generation programmes should be launched in the region because there is no scope for heavy industries etc. like other parts of India. Local participation must be considered at the time of policy framing.

Notes

1. The population of India includes the estimated population of entire Kachchh district, Morvi, Maliya-Miyana and Wankaner talukas of Rajkot district, Jodiya taluka of Jamnagar district of Gujarat state and entire Kinnaur district of Himachal Pradesh while the literacy data are not included where population enumeration of Census of India, 2001, could not be conducted due to natural calamities.
2. The population figures for Jammu and Kashmir have been interpolated for the year 1991 as the 1991 Census not be conducted in the state due to disturbed conditions.
3. The literacy rates for the year 1981 relate to the population aged five years and above while the year 1991 and 2001 relate to the population aged seven years and above.

3

Uttarakhand Himalaya: Geo-Physical Environment

3.1 Physiography

Uttarakhand Himalaya comprises all the five latitudinal physiographic-geological zones – the Tarai-Bhabar, the Siwalik with duns, the Lesser Himalaya, the Great Himalaya and the Trans Himalaya (Figs. 3.1 and 3.2).

The northern fringe of Indo-Gangetic plains, waterlogged in older times, is known as Tarai. Due to the availability of fertile soil, hot climate coupled with abundant water, this 10-25 km wide, once densely forested Tarai belt has been the home land of Tharus, Bukshas and Gujjars, and is largely reclaimed for agriculture. Due to introduction of new agrarian techniques by the enterprising hardworking refuges from Pakistan and Bangladesh, retired army personnel and freedom fighters of Uttarakhand, the Tarai today is one of the most developed parts of the country. In the Tarai, Bhabar, Dun and adjoining Siwalik belts, there are about 13% of rural settlements and 60% of urban centers including Dehradun, Rishikesh, Kotdwar, Kalagarh, Ramnagar, Kashipur, Haldwani-cum-Rathgodam, Tanakpur, Khatima, Rudrapur, Sitarganj, Gadarpur, Kichchha,

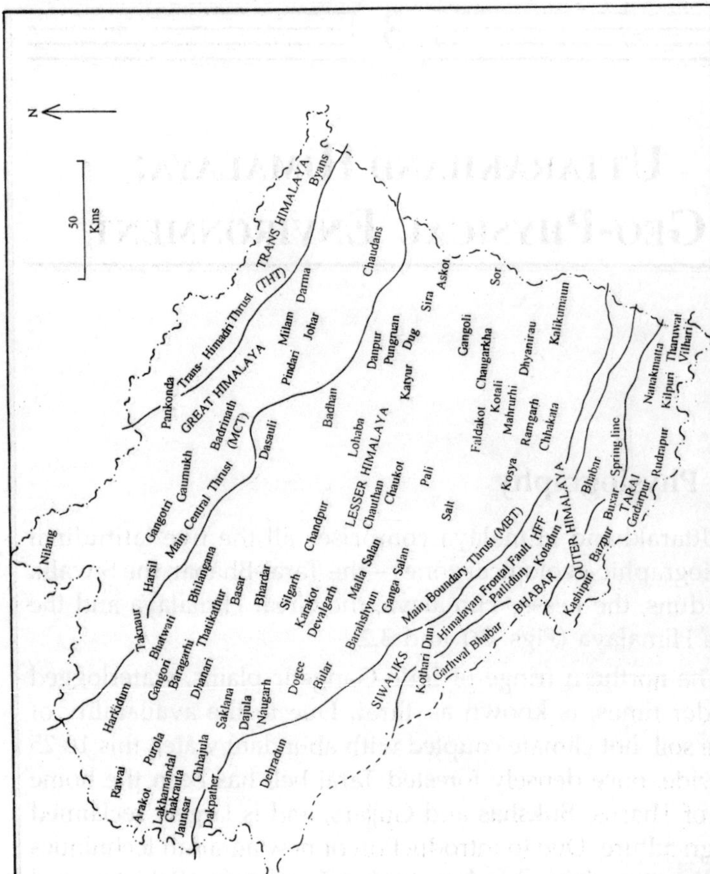

Fig. 3.1. Physiographic Divisions of Uttarakhand.

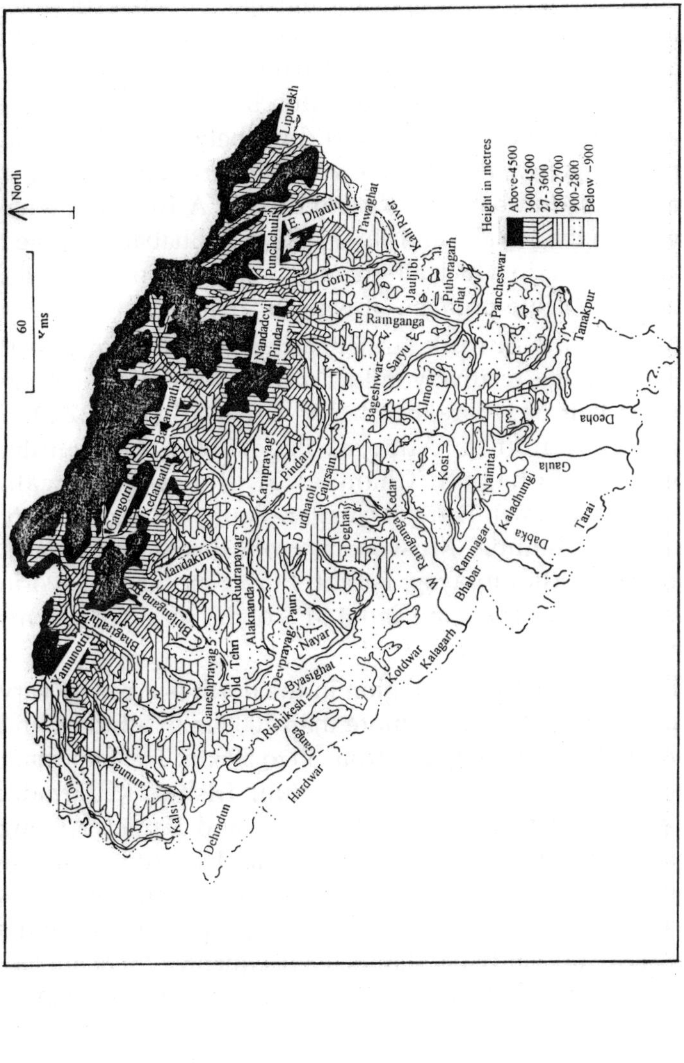

Fig. 3.2. Relief Map of Uttarakhand.

Bazpur, Jaspur, Pantnagar (Nagla) etc. There are several reservoirs Nanaksagar, Bahgul, Haripura, Tumeria and Kalagarh.

With the altitude varying from 700 to 1200 m, the Siwalik, like the Bhabar region, is sparsely inhabited because of thick vegetal cover and water scarcity. The gravel filled, almost plain latitudinal areas in the Siwalik domain are known as *Duns*. There are five duns, namely Dehradun between Yamuna and Ganga, Chaukhamba and Kothari duns between Ganga and Western Ramganga, Patlidun between Western Ramganga and Kosi and Kotadun between Kosi and Baur. A 10-20 km wide belt between the Siwalik and Tarai known as Bhabar, is formed by coarse gravels in which all streams disappear. Consequently, the belt faces acute problem of water scarcity.

North of the Siwalik stretches the 70-km wide Lesser Himalaya having relatively milder terrain. This is the densely populated belt of Uttarakhand. The Urban centers (37%) of Dwarahat, Ranikhet, Almora, Bageshwar, Dharchula, Pithoragarh, Lohaghat, Champawat, Bhimtal, Bhawali, Nainital, Lansdown, Narendranagar, Pauri, Srinagar, Tehri, Uttarkashi, Chamba, Mussoorie, Gopeshwar, Joshimath, Karnaprayag, Rudraprayag, Barkot, Purola etc. are located in Lesser Himalaya. There are about 81% of the rural settlements in the Lesser Himalaya.

The Great Himalayan region in the north is a belt of very high peaks from 3000 m to more than 7000 m in altitude, and of glaciers. It ranges in width from 30 to 50 km. The important peaks include Nandadevi, Panchchuli, Trishul, Kedarnath, Chaukhamba, Badrinath, Bandarpunch and Kamet. Among the glacier Pindari, Milám, Gangotri and Khatling are the important ones. The harsh and rigorous climatic conditions together with extremely rugged topography are perhaps responsible for scanty habitation. Consequently, there are less than 70 seasonal settlements in the river valleys and *bugyals* (alpine pasture).

The Trans-Himalaya belt is 40 km wide. This is a rain shadow zone as southeastern monsoon clouds cannot cross the Great Himalaya. The belt is scantily populated, there being just 20-30 temporary villages of the Bhotia tribes.

3.2 Geology

From the geological point of view, the Uttarakhand or Kumaun Lesser Himalaya is divided into five lithotectonic units (Figs. 3.1 and 3.3). These units are demarcated by several thrusts and faults. Most of these faults/thrusts are active. The brief description of the geology/structure is based on Valdiya (1980 and 1988).

3.2.1 The Outer Himalaya

The foothill belt of Kumaun Lesser Himalaya is made of sandstone, mudstone and subordinate conglomerates of the Middle Miocene to Early Pleistocene age. The Lower Siwalik consists of fined grained calcareous subgrawacks and sub litharenites alternating with dominant horizons of maroon mudstone and rare paraconglomerates while the Middle Siwalik consists of predominant coarse-grained sub litharentic and subordinate paraconglomerate. The Upper Siwalik sediment comprising boulder conglomerate with maroon mudstone and sandstone were deposited largely by braided rivers. Himalayan Front Fault (HFF) separates Siwalik from the Bhabar. The gravel filled synclinal valleys are known as *Duns* – Dehradun, Chaukhamba, Kothari, Patli and Kotadun. It includes two lithotectonic units – (1) Tarai and Bhabar, and (2) Siwalik.

3.2.2 The Lesser Himalaya

Lying between the MBT in the south and MCT in the north, the Lesser Himalayan terrain is made of three lithotectonic units:

1. The autochthonous succession of the Precambrian strata forming the larger part of the inner belt.
2. Late Precambrian to early Paleozoic sedimentary rocks formation forming the Krol Nappe includes slates, phylites, sandstone, and limestone.

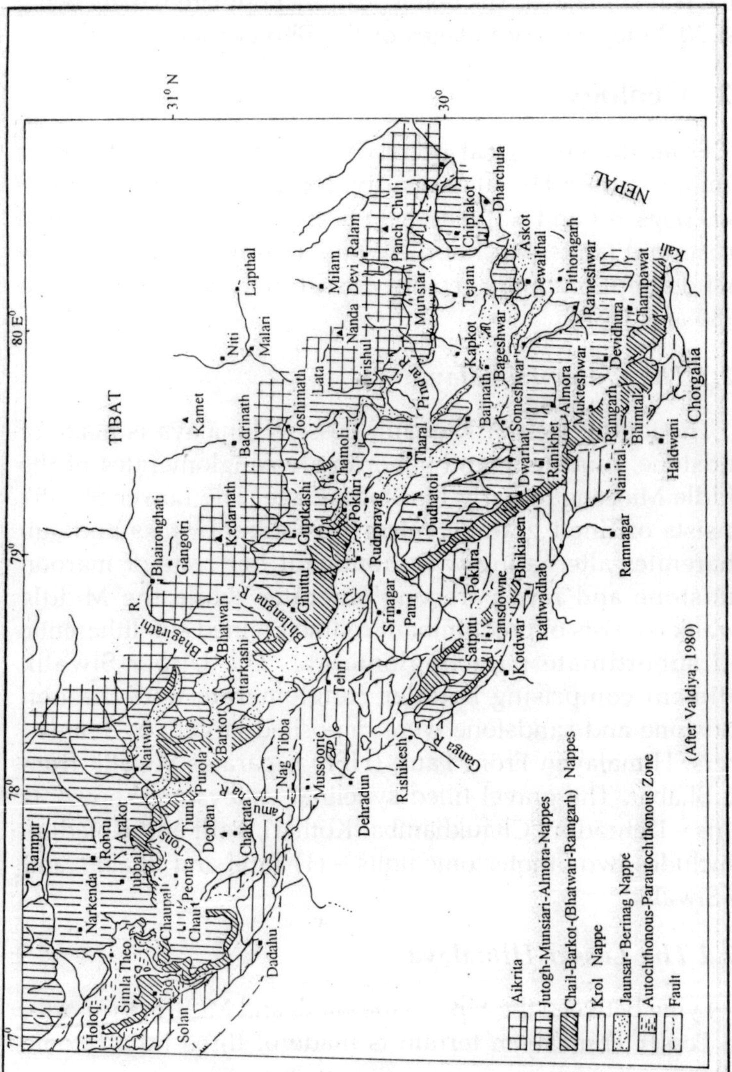

Fig. 3.3. Structural Map of Uttarakhand.

Table 3.1. Lithotectonic Succession in Uttarakhand Himalaya

Northern Belt	*Southern Belt*
Jungbwa Ultrabascis	
------ Jungbwa Thrust ------	
Kiogarhophiolitic Melange	
------ Kiogarh Thrust ------	
Tethyan Succession	
(Late Precambrian – Late Cetaceous	
--- Trans-Himadri (Malari) Thrust ---	
Vaikrita Group	
(Precambrian)	
--- Main Central (Vaikarita) Thrust ---	Almora Group
Munsyari Formation	(with 550 ± 50 m.y. granite)
(Early Precambrian)	
----- Munsyari Thrust -----	----- Almora Thrust -----
(Schuppen Zone)	Ramgarh Group
Bhatwari – Barkot Formations	(with 1900 ± 100 m.y. porphyroids)
----- Bhatwari – Barkot Thrust -----	----- Ramgarh Thrust -----
Berinag Formation	Krol Succession
(Precambrian)	(Late Precambrian–Lower Cambrian)
	Subhathu Fm
	Unidentified Paleocene (Singtali) [Sirmur Group
	Tal Fm, Krol Fm, Blaini Fm [Mussoorie Group
	Nagthat Fm, Chandpur Fm [Jaunsar Group
----- Berinag Thrust -----	---- Krol or Main Boundary Thrust ----
Tejam Gr. [Mandali Fm., Daoban Fm	Siwalik Group
	(Late Tertiary)
Damtha Gr. [Rautgara Fm., Chakrata Fm.	
(Precambrian)	
Base not exposed	----- Himalayan Front Fault -----
	Ganga plain with Bhabar Fan
	(Quaternary Recent)

Source: Valdiya (1980 and 1988).

3. The Precambrian metamorphic injected was granite bodies.

In summing up there are seven main lithological groups namely, Krol succession, Ramgarh group, Almora group, Damtha – Tejam group, Bhatwari – Barkot formation, Berinag formation, and Munsyari formation. (Table 3.1 & Fig. 3.3).

3.2.3 The Great Himalaya

The Great Himalaya is made of high grade metamorphic – the Vaikrita group of Precambrian age and intruded extensively by mid Tertiary granite. However, Jhingran referred it Central Crystalline Zone (Jhingran, 1981).

3.2.4 The Trans Himalaya

Trans Himadri Thrust – separates the Trans Himalaya from the Great Himalaya. The rock formations are shattered mylonolized or otherwise complexly folded.

3.3 Drainage

Uttarakhand is drained by the network of the Ganga and the Kali systems comprising the Yamuna, the Ganga, and the Kali (Sharda) rivers (Fig. 3.4).

The Yamuna originates from the Yamunotri hot spring and Saptrishikund on the southwestern slope of the Bandarpunch ridge and flows through the district of Uttarkashi and Dehradun. The Tons is the largest river in respect of volume of water flowing. Bhagirathi and Alaknanda join at Devprayag to make the Ganga river. The Bhilangana is the main tributary of the Bhagirathi which rises from Khatling glacier. Western Dahuli originates at Untadhura and Niti Pass on the Indo-Tibet water divide, and joins the Vishnuganga at Vishnuprayag. Saraswati, emanating near Mana Pass, makes the headwaters of the Alaknanda. Pindar (originating from Pindari glacier) and Mandakini (rising in the Kedarnath ridge) are the main tributaries of the Alaknanda. Nayar joining the Ganga from the west at Byasighat, drains the Dudhatoli-Pauri Ridge.

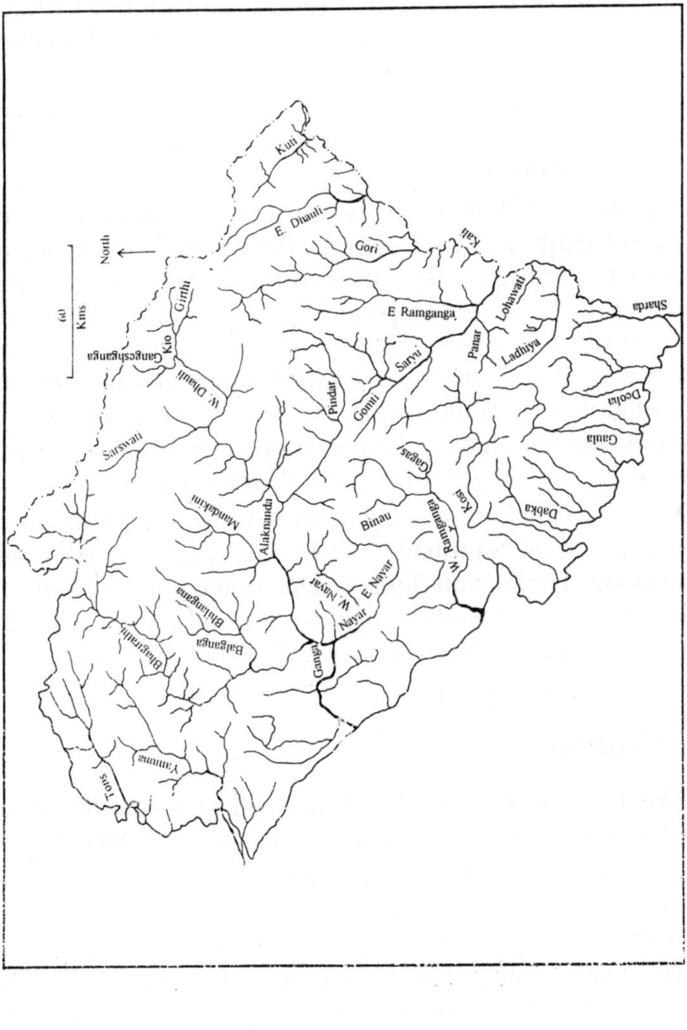

Fig. 3.4. Drainage Map of Uttarakhand.

Kali is the largest river in Kumaun both in respect of volume of water as well as extent of the catchment area. It is also largest river in Uttarakhand in respect of length. The Kali originates at Kalapani near the Lipulekh Pass and is fed by Kuti, Eastern Dhauli, Gori, Saryu, Lohawati and Ladhiya rivers. Gori emanates from the Milam glacier and Eastern Ramganga from Namik glacier. Eastern Ramganga and Panar are the principal tributaries of the Saryu. Saryu joins the Kali at Pancheshwar. Entering the plain at Baramedeo the Kali known as Sharda river.

The Western Ramganga rises from the northest slope of Dudhatoli ridge in Pauri district. Binau the head water of Western Ramganga, takes its rise from the Binsar spring located on the southern slope of Dudhatoli range. It joins the Masangaddi and Western Ramganga at Deghat and Kedar respectively. Rising from the Bhatkot ridge, Gagas joins the W. Ramganga at Bhikiasain. The Kosi river rises on the southern slope of Bhatkot – Kausani range and leave Kumaun near Sarkara eventually to join the Western Ramganga.

Minor rivers like Song, Khoh, Rispana, Dhela, Dabka, Baur, Bhakhara, Gaula, Nandhaur and Deoha, drain the outer belt of the Lesser Himalayan domain. Due to the porous nature of Bhabar areas these rivulets became dry and reappear in the Tarai region where these are checked in the form of artificial reservoirs for multipurpose.

3.4 Climate

The Tarai-Bhabar and low-lying valleys below 800 m of elevation have hot and humid climate. Between 800-1200 m elevation, it is subtropical, temperate from 1200 to 2000 m, cool temperate between 2400-3000 m elevation cold temperate; and above 3000 m of elevation very cold alpine.

The mean temperature in the January is about 21° C in the submountain belt of Tarai, Bhabar and Duns while 8° C in the inner valleys. June register highest temperatures – around 40° C in Tarai-Bhabar and Dun belts, 24° C in the Lesser Himalayan domain and 15 – 20° C at higher places. About

80% of the total rainfall occurs in the monsoon months alone. The average annual rainfall is 150 cm in the Tarai-Bhabar and Dun belts, while the Nainital hills receives the highest i.e. 250 cm., then decreasing north-wards in the inner Lesser Himalaya where the average annual rainfall is only 90 cm. The Trans-Himalayan region falls in the rain shadow zone, because the southeast monsoon clouds cannot cross the Great Himalaya.

3.5 Vegetation

The tree line lies at an altitude of about 4200 m. The forests of the region have been classified as follows (Champion and Seth, 1968):

1. Tropical Moist Deciduous Forests
2. Tropical Dry Deciduous Forests
3. Sub-tropical Pine Forests
4. Sub-tropical Dry Evergreen Forests
5. Himalayan Moist Temperate Forests
6. Himalayan Dry Temperate Forests
7. Sub-Apline Forests
8. Moist Alpine Forests
9. Dry Alpine Shrubs

3.6 Soil

A complete soil survey of the Uttarakhand Himalaya has not been carried out so far. Based on the available data, it becomes difficult to determine the remarkable characteristics of the soil. The foothill soil near Dehradun show that the soils are loam to clay-loam in texture and acidic in nature. In Ranikhet area four broad soil groups have been identified – red loam, brown forest soil, podzolic soil and meadow soil (Ghildyal, 1981). On the basis of altitude, lithology, landscape, slope aspect, gradient, vegetation, drainage and field work, the soil of Kotadun, south western part of Kumaun Himalaya is classified into seven groups – loamous soil, conglomeratic sandy soil, stony hilly soil, crushed slaty soil, hill sandy soil, podzolic soil and rocky thin regolithic soil (Pant, 1994).

4

UTTARAKHAND HIMALAYA: ECO-CULTURAL ENVIRONMENT

In broad sense, the eco-cultural environment of a geographical unit include all human activities regarding to agriculture, floriculture, sericulture, pisciculture, settlement, demographic features, livestock, developmental indicators, fairs, festivals, songs, dances etc. which vary from one place to another. Some of these aspects are considered in the present study.

4.1 Demographic Setting

Demographic profile concerns with the growth, distribution, sex ratio, literacy, occupation etc. The population study of any region is necessary from the view point of economic welfare scheme. One plan must be framed in the light of past and present demographic features. Development planning gets changed on account of the requirements of growing population. Varied environment, the distribution pattern and growth of population also vary from one place to another. Physical environment is the most dominant aspect to permit or restrict man's activities.

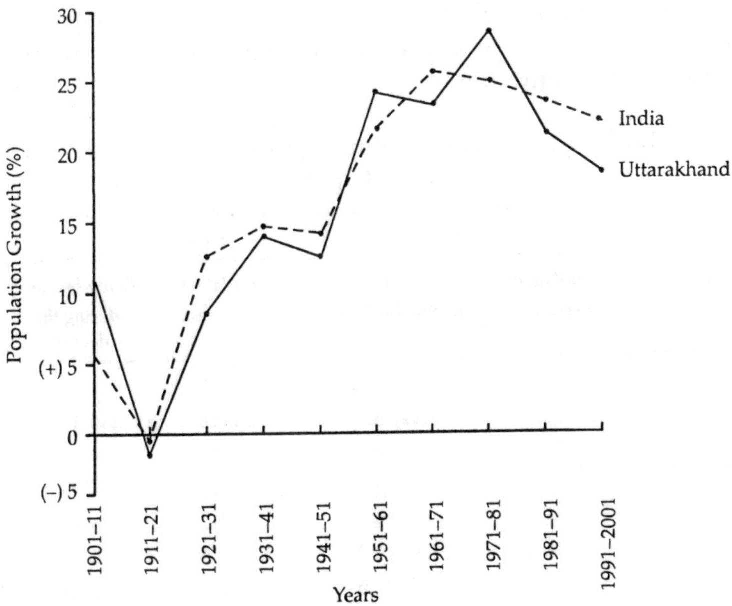

Fig. 4.1. Population Growth in Uttarakhand and India.

4.1.1 Population Distribution and Growth

The population distribution and growth pattern, considered as they are by environment differ from one area to another. The population of Uttarakhand is concentrated in Tarai, Bhabar, Duns and lower levels of valleys of the Lesser Himalayan rivers. According to the 2001 census, the 70.35 lakh people of Uttarakhand live in 15117 villages and 64 towns. The density of population in 2001 varies from 37 persons/km^2 in Uttarkashi district to 424 persons/km^2 in Dehradun district. In 1991, it was 30 and 329 persons/km^2 respectively (Table 4.3 and 4.4). Total population of Uttarakhand increased 18.72% during the period of 1991 to 2001 compared to 21.45% in the whole country (Table 4.1 and Fig. 4.1).

About 57.19% villages have population less than 200, (31.37%) 200-499, (8.70%) 500-999, (2.19%) 1000-1999, (0.48%) 2000-4999 and only 0.07% villages have more than 5000 people (Table 4.2). The large size of settlements are in the district Nainital and Dehradun.

Table 4.1. Growth of Population in India and Uttarakhand, 1901–2001

	India		*Uttarakhand*	
Census Year	*Population (in crores)*	*% inc. (+)/dec. (–) during the decades*	*Population (in crores)*	*% inc. (+)/dec. during the decades*
1901	23.8	–	0.16	–
1911	25.2	(+) 5.7	0.18	(+) 11.0
1921	25.1	(–) 0.3	0.18	(–) 0.6
1931	27.9	(+) 11.0	0.19	(+) 8.3
1941	31.9	(+) 14.2	0.22	(+) 13.7
1951	36.1	(+) 13.3	0.25	(+) 12.3
1961	43.9	(+) 21.5	0.31	(+) 23.3
1971	54.8	(+) 24.8	0.38	(+)23.0
1981	68.5	(+) 24.7	0.48	(+) 26.5
1991	84.6	(+) 23.5	0.59	(+) 21.5
2001	102.7	(+) 21.35	0.70	(+) 18.7
1901–2001	(+) 78.9	(+) 330.8	(+) 0.54	(+) 326.4

Source: Anon, 1991(a), (b), 2001; Pant, 1995a and 1996a.

The number of urban centers (census town), which was 18 in 1901, rose to 76 in 2001 where 24.51% of the population is concentrated. The Uttarakhand region has registered tremendous growth of population (Figure 4.1). There is 326.4% increase during the period of 1901 to 2001 compared to 330.8% in the whole country (Table 4.1).

4.1.2 Gender Composition

The average male-female ratio in 1991 was 976 females per one thousand Males – 851 in Dehradun and 1128 in Almora

Table 4.2. Size of Rural Settlements in Uttarakhand, 1981

District/ Region	*No. of Settlements*	*No. of Inhabited Settlements*	*Population Size (% of Inhabited Settlements)*					
			Below 200	*200–499*	*500–999*	*1000–1999*	*2000–4999*	*Above 5000*
Uttarkashi	681	669	48.28	40.06	10.16	1.35	0.15	–
Chamoli	1,632	1,516	57.26	34.10	7.85	0.79	–	–
Tehri	2,020	1,953	51.61	38.61	8.55	1.23	–	–
Dehradun	763	743	46.57	29.74	12.38	7.00	3.10	1.21
Pauri	3,573	3,237	69.86	25.39	4.17	0.46	0.12	–
Pithoragarh	2,243	2,174	63.89	27.55	7.13	1.20	0.23	–
Almora	3,165	3,019	56.38	33.32	9.04	1.26	–	–
Nainital	1,856	1,806	41.42	30.73	16.95	8.58	2.21	0.11
Uttarakhand	**15,973**	**15,117**	**57.19**	**31.37**	**8.70**	**2.19**	**0.48**	**0.07**

Source: Pant, 1995a and 1996a.

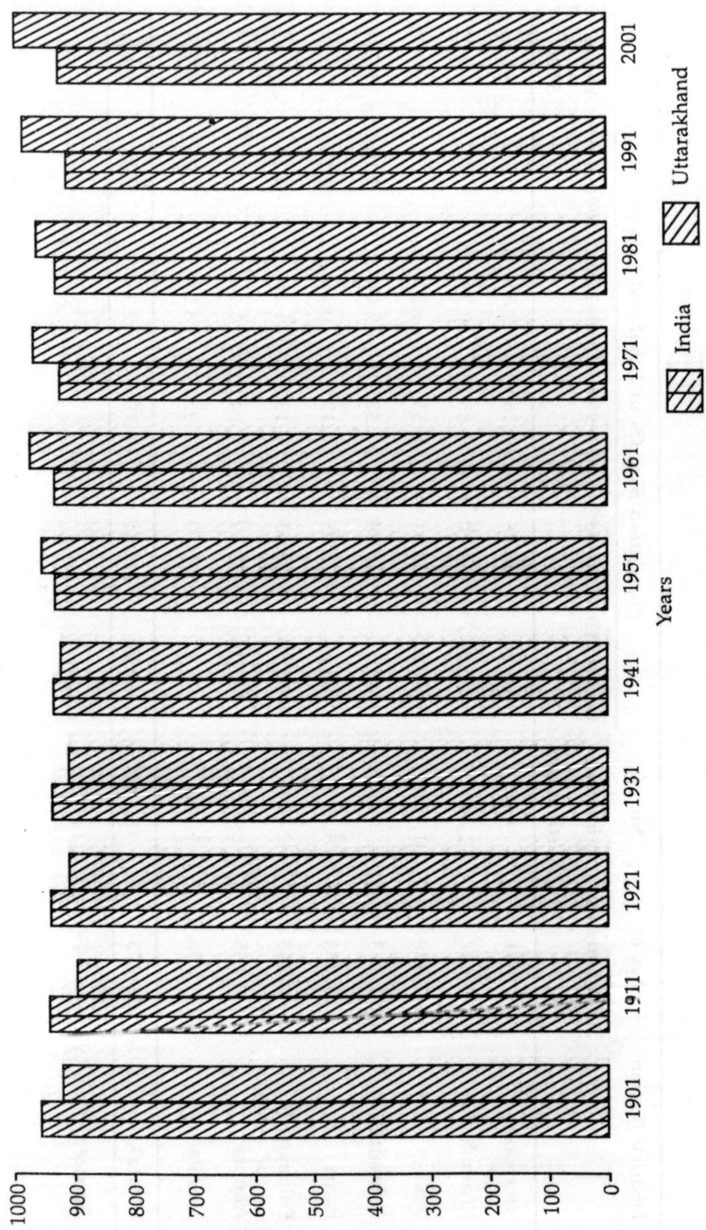

Fig. 4.2. Sex Ratio in Uttarakhand and India.

Table [illegible].3. Districtwise Population Variation, Density, Sex Ratio and Literacy of Uttarakhand

District/ Region	*Total (T) Rural (R) Urban (U) Male/Female (M/F)*	*Population Variation (%) (1901–1991)*	*Population Density (persons/km²)*			*Sex Ratio (Females/1000 Males)*		*Literacy (%)*		
			(1971)	*(1981)*	*(1991)*	*(1981)*	*(1991)*	*(1971)*	*(1981)*	*(1991)*
1	**2**	**3**	**4**	**5**	**6**	**7**	**8**	**9**	**10**	**11**
	T	(+) 243.5	14	24	30	881	928	20.04	28.92	47.23
Uttarkashi	R	(+) 218.8	17	22	28	909	950	20.29	26.21	44.50
	U	(+) 540.7	502	758	1006	571	684	63.22	65:20	80.93
	M/F	–	–	–	–	–	–	37.0/5.4	46.3/9.2	68.74/23.57
	T	(+) 203.2	32	41	50	1093	1059	28.67	37.46	61.08
Chamoli	R	(+) 177.7	31	37	46	1090	1100	27.48	35.16	68.95
	U	(+) 163.5	406	389	547	623	695	56.04	63.87	81.42
	M/F	–	–	–	–	–	–	48.9/4.9	57.4/9.4	82.01/40.37
	T	(+) 187.9	90	113	131	1081	1073	19.29	27.89	48.38
Tehri	R	(+) 171.4	88	109	125	1119	1115	18.08	26.20	46.46
	U	(+) 362.3	222	412	588	555	560	63.43	67.07	78.41
	M/F	–	–	–	–	–	–	36.4/4.9	48.0/9.4	72.10/26.41
	T	(+) 471.8	187	247	332	811	851	43.74	52.58	69.50
Dehradun	R	(+) 262.6	105	134	177	839	878	27.20	38.84	57.34
	U	(+) 1203.1	1648	2157	2599	783	825	62.34	66.97	81.04
	M/F	–	–	–	–	–	–	51.7/33.4	61.1/42.0	77.95/59.26

Contd.

1	2	3	4	5	6	7	8	9	10	11
	T	(+) 134.3	102	116	126	1091	1112	32.00	41.06	63.35
Pauri	R	(+) 110.9	96	107	112	1147	1184	30.13	38.46	63.85
	U	(+) 1051.4	564	911	1199	682	707	59.79	64.88	76.11
	M/F	–	–	–	–	–	–	49.3/16.5	56.3/27.1	82.46/49.44
	T	(+) 236.2	43	55	64	1014	1030	34.87	39.08	59.01
Pithoragarh	R	(+) 207.6	42	52	59	1035	1053	30.74	37.37	56.88
	U	(+) 253.0	1846	757	1210	717	784	60.32	68.37	84.32
	M/F	–	–	–	–	–	–	48.2/12.7	58.1/20.3	79.44/38.37
	T	(+) 153.4	107	141	155	1081	1128	28.08	37.76	58.66
Almora	R	(+) 183.0	102	133	146	1118	1151	25.91	35.21	56.62
	U	(+) 300.6	1470	1262	1421	649	817	67.57	75.69	86.36
	M/F	–	–	–	–	–	–	46.3/12.3	56.7/20.3	79.96/39.60
	T	(+) 3180.5	116	168	227	841	873	31.94	37.81	56.52
Nainital	R	(+) 285.08	91	123	156	848	887	27.44	33.24	52.55
	U	(+) 1178.6	3843	3769	4032	821	841	44.77	49.86	64.62
	M/F	–	–	–	–	–	–	41.3/20.2	46.8/27.1	67.88/43.19
	T	**(+) 257.6**	**75**	**95**	**116**	**959**	**976**	**31.02**	**39.29**	**59.58**
Uttarakhand	**R**	**(+) 198.0**	**64**	**78**	**92**	**1009**	**1027**	**26.40**	**34.39**	**55.22**
	U	**(+) 1205.4**	**1422**	**1639**	**2107**	**764**	**809**	**57.86**	**61.17**	**74.78**
	M/F	**–**	**–**	**–**	**–**	**–**	**–**	**45.6/16.0**	**53.8/24.1**	**75.51/42.87**

Source: Anon, 1981a and 1991a.

Note: Literacy rates for 1991 relate to the population aged 7 years and above.

Table 4.4. Districtwise Demographic Profile of Uttaranchal State, 2001

Sl. No.	*Districts/ State*	*Area (Km²)*	*Inhibated villages (No.)*	*Development Block (No.)*	*Tehsil (No.)*	*Statutory Town Area(No.)*	*Total Population*		
							Person	*Male*	*Female*
1	2	3	4	5	6	7	8	9	10
1.	Uttrakashi	8016	678	06	04	03	294179	151599	142580
2.	Chamoli	7614	1186	09	06	06	369198	183033	186165
3.	Rudraprayag	1891	660	03	02	02	227461	107425	120036
4.	Tehri	4080	1742	09	05	07	604608	294842	309766
5.	Dehradun	3088	726	06	04	14	1279083	675549	603534
6.	Pauri	5400	3174	15	06	06	696851	331138	365713
7.	Pithoragarh	7100	1551	08	05	04	462149	227592	234557
8.	Champawat	1781	623	04	01	04	224461	110916	113545
9.	Almora	3083	2139	11	03	04	630446	293576	336870
10.	Bageshwar	2302	885	03	02	01	249453	118202	131251
11.	Nainital	3860	1095	08	04	08	762912	400336	362576
12.	U. Singh Nagar	2908	687	07	04	17	1234548	649020	585528
13.	Hardwar	2360	503	06	03	10	1444213	773173	671040
	Uttaranchal	**53483**	**15669**	**95**	**49**	**86**	**8479562**	**4316401**	**4163161**

Contd.

Sl. No.	Districts/ State	% of Total Population	Rank (No.)	Growth (%) 1991-2001	Density (P/km²)	Sex Ratio (Female/1000 Males)	Literates (%)		
							Person	Male	Female
1	2	11	12	13	14	15	16	17	18
1.	Uttrakashi	3.47	10	22.72	37	941	66.58	84.52	47.48
2.	Chamoli	4.35	09	13.51	48	1017	76.23	89.89	63.00
3.	Rudraprayag	2.68	12	13.44	120	1117	74.23	90.73	59.98
4.	Tehri	7.13	07	16.15	148	1051	67.04	85.62	49.76
5.	Dehradun	15.08	02	24.71	414	893	78.96	85.87	71.22
6.	Pauri	8.22	05	3.87	129	1104	77.99	91.47	66.14
7.	Pithoragarh	5.45	08	10.92	65	1031	76.48	90.57	63.14
8.	Champawat	2.65	13	17.56	126	1024	71.11	88.13	54.75
9.	Almora	7.43	06	3.14	205	1147	74.53	90.15	61.43
10.	Bageshwar	2.94	11	9.21	108	1110	71.94	88.56	57.45
11.	Nainital	9.00	04	32.88	198	906	79.60	87.39	70.98
12.	U. Singh Nagar	14.56	03	27.79	424	902	65.76	76.20	54.16
13.	Hardwar	17.04	01	26.30	612	868	64.60	75.06	52.60
	Uttaranchal	**100.00**	–	**19.20**	**159**	**964**	**72.28**	**84.10**	**60.26**

Source: Anon, 2001.

(Table 4.3 and Fig. 4.2). The number of females in the urban dominated (Dehradun and Nainital) districts are fewer than that of rural-based districts (Chamoli, Pauri, Tehri, Uttarkashi, Pithoragarh and Almora). Most probably it is due to the out migration of men from the hilly villages.

4.1.3 Pyramidal Age Structure

More than 38% of the population belongs the age group below 14 years at the base of the population pyramid and 7.0% of the people are above 60 years in age. Of these 54.30% are in the group of working age (15-59) and 45.0% belong to the age group of dependents. All districts exhibit nearly the same trend (Table 4.5 and Fig. 4.3).

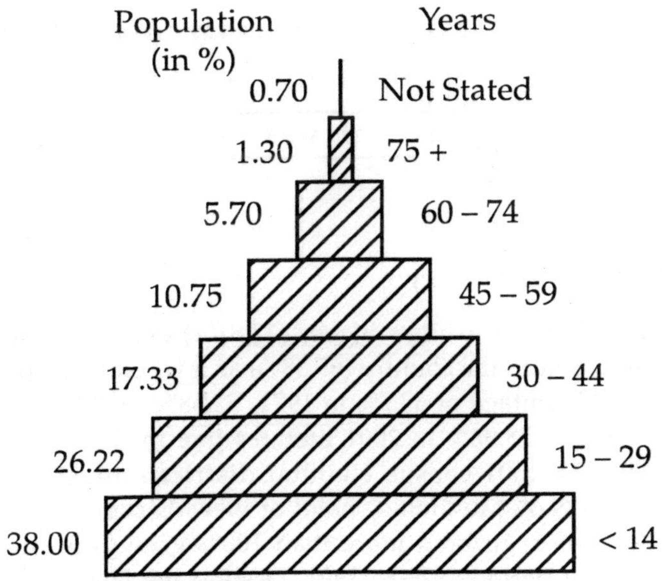

Fig. 4.3. Age Structure in Uttarakhand, 1991.

Table 4.5. Population of Uttarakhand in Various Age Groups, 1991

District/ Region	*Years*							
	Below 14	*15-29*	*30-44*	*45-59*	*60-74*	*Above 75*	*N.S.*	*Total*
Uttarkashi	36.99	26.57	17.39	11.09	5.53	1.49	0.94	100
Pauri	37.46	26.05	15.86	11.41	6.85	1.52	0.85	100
Chamoli	38.34	25.85	16.46	11.86	5.50	1.31	0.68	100
Tehri	39.49	25.26	15.92	10.89	6.77	1.31	0.36	100
Dehradun	34.94	28.75	19.28	10.45	4.94	1.05	0.59	100
Almora	38.87	23.84	16.31	12.13	6.96	1.48	0.41	100
Nainital	39.32	26.80	17.97	9.12	4.50	1.21	1.08	100
Pithoragarh	37.98	24.95	17.46	11.73	6.17	1.38	0.33	100
Uttarakhand	**38.00**	**26.22**	**17.33**	**10.75**	**5.70**	**1.30**	**0.70**	**100**

Source: Anon 1991a.

N.S.: Not stated.

4.1.4 State of Literacy

Uttarakhand exhibits higher (73.81%) degree of literacy as compared to the country (65.38%) as a whole in 2001. The largest percentage of 43.7% in 1971, 52.58% in 1981, 58.55% in 1991 and 78.96% in 2001 literates live in the Dehradun district. In 2001 census Nainital district ranked in first position (79.6%) in literacy point of view. Excepting Almora all districts registered more than 100% growth in literacy during the period 1971 to 1991. Despite the fast growth in literacy, 26.19% of the total population is still illiterate – 38.32% of female is illiterate in 2001 (Tables 4.3 and 4.4 and Figure 4.4).

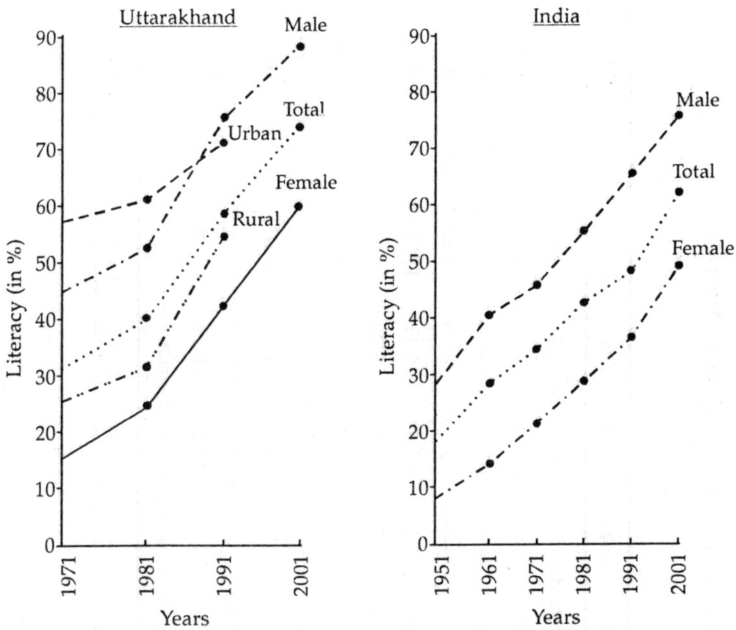

Fig. 4.4. Literacy in Uttarakhand and India.

4.1.5 Level of Urbanisation

The state of socio-economic development of any society is often viewed by the degree of urbanisation attained by the particular society in a specified space and time. The growth of urban population in Uttarakhand has been steadily upward since 1901 (Table 4.6). The percentage of urban population of the region was 21.70% in 1991. It is remarkably remained low in Uttarkashi (7.20%), Pauri (11.89%), Chamoli (8.91%), Tehri (5.67%), Almora (6.40%) and Pithoragarh (7.44%). Table 4.6 reveals the percentage of urban population of Uttarakhand as a whole was 5.91% in 1901, 6.70% in 1911 and 7.29% in 1921 white it decreased 6.70% in 1931, otherwise it shows the increasing trend at every decades (Fig. 4.5). The percentage

Table 4.6. Level of Urbanisation in Uttarakhand, 1901–2001

District/Region	*1901*	*1911*	*1921*	*1931*	*1941*	*1951*	*1961*	*1971*	*1981*	*1991*	*2001*
Uttarkashi	------------ Did not exist as a seperate district ------------						2.18	4.10	6.95	7.20	7.79
Chamoli	------------ do ------------							4.17	8.01	8.91	13.43
Rudraprayag	------------ do ------------										1.20
Tehri	------------ do ------------					2.33	2.18	2.65	4.13	5.67	9.67
Dehradun	22.23	27.21	31.30	28.01	35.26	47.44	46.11	47.08	48.86	50.26	52.94
Pauri	2.49	2.98	2.97	1.93	2.75	4.25	5.70	6.30	9.82	11.89	12.94
Pithoragarh	------------ Did not exist as a separate district ------------							2.87	5.54	7.44	12.14
Champawat	------------ do ------------										14.58
Almora	3.67	4.36	3.17	3.24	3.57	4.27	4.30	6.07	6.28	6.40	
Bageshwar	------------ Did not exist as a separate district ------------										3.13
Nainital	12.19	12.87	16.35	17.30	23.63	22.30	19.53	22.13	27.49	32.66	35.36
Udham Singh Nagar	------------ Did not exist as a separate district ------------										32.65
Uttarakhand	**5.91**	**6.70**	**7.29**	**6.70**	**8.43**	**11.68**	**12.07**	**14.69**	**18.30**	**21.70**	**24.51**

Source: Anon, 1981(a), 1991(a) and 2001.

of urban population of the region is 24.51 in 2001. Maximum 52.94% urban population in Dehradun district and minimum 1.2% in Rudraprayag district. Number of urban centers from 1901 to 2001 are presented table 4.7.

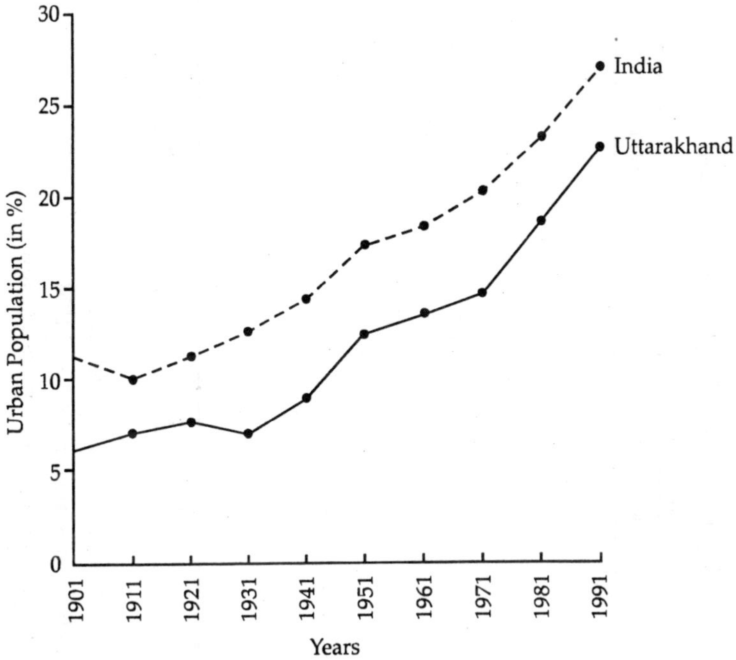

Fig. 4.5. Urban Population in Uttarakhand and India.

4.1.6 Occupational Structure

The working population, which was 45.61% in 1961, declined to 36.36% in 1991. On the other hand the tertiary sector showed increasing trend, partly due to out migration from rural to urban centers for mostly white collar jobs. The percentage of main workers in the total population recorded higher in Uttarakhand (36.33%) compared to the country

Table 4.7. Number of Towns[1] in Uttarakhand

District/Region	*2001*	*1991*	*1981*	*1971*	*1961*	*1951*	*1941*	*1931*	*1921*	*1911*	*1901*
Uttarkashi	03	3	3	1	1	1*	–	–	–	–	–
Chamoli	06	8	7	3	–	–	–	–	–	–	–
Rudraprayag	02	–	–	–	–	–	–	–	–	–	–
Tehri***	07	4	5	4	3	5	–	–	–	–	–
Dehradun	14	16	11	9	8	8	7	7	7	7	6
Pauri	06	8	8	6	6	5	3	3	4	3	3
Pithoragarh	04	5	5	1	–	1**	–	–	–	–	–
Champawat	04	–	–	–	–	–	–	–	–	–	–
Almora	04	5	5	4	3	3	3	3	2	2	2
Bageshwar	01	–	–	–	–	–	–	–	–	–	–
Nainital	08	25	18	9	8	7	8	8	8	6	7
U. S. Nagar	17	–	–	–	–	–	–	–	–	–	–
Uttarakhand	**76**	**74**	**62**	**37**	**29**	**30**	**21**	**21**	**21**	**18**	**18**

Source: Anon, 1981a and 1991b.

Notes: 1. Total Statutory Units. * – Uttarkashi T. A. which fell in Tehri in 1951.

** – Pithoragarh T. A. which fell in Almora in 1941 and 1951.

*** – Tehri district was princely state from 1901 to 1941 Censuses.

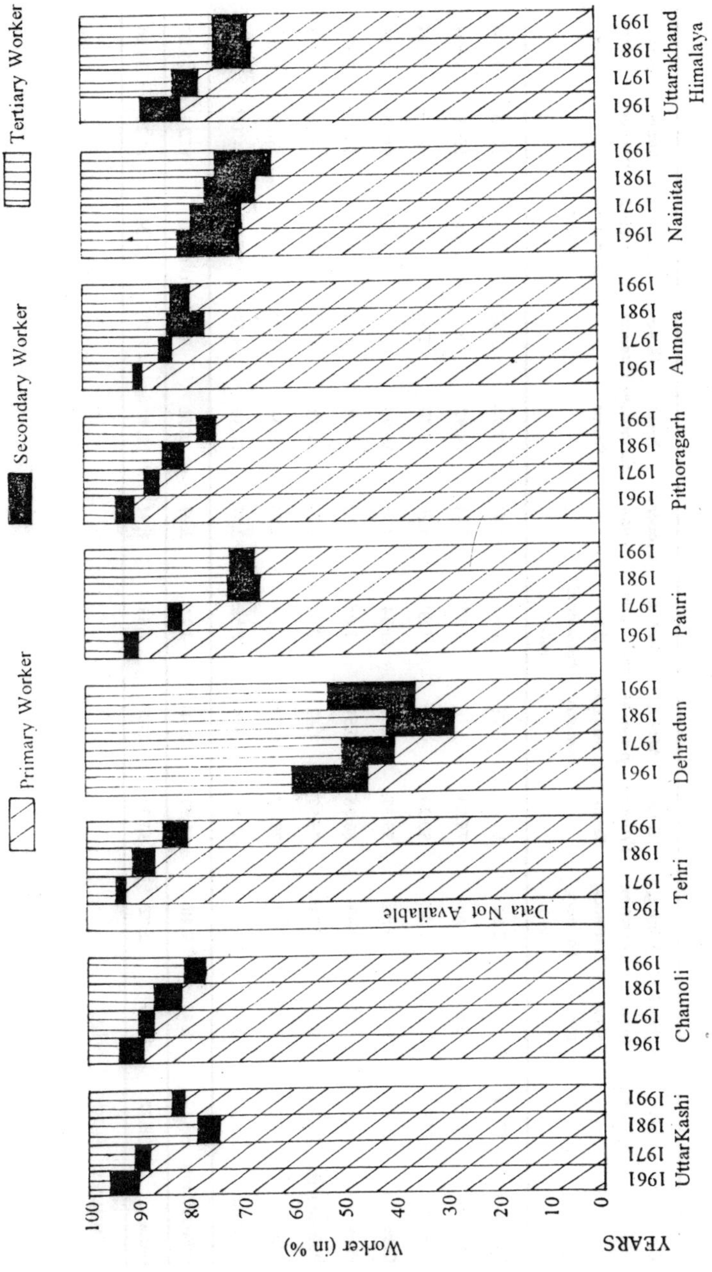

Fig. 4.6. Occupational Structure in Uttarakhand.

Table 4.8. Districtwise Occupational Structure in Uttarakhand, 1991

District	Culti-vators	Agricul-tural Labou-rers	Mining, Quarring Livestock, Forestry, etc.	Total Primary Sector	Maf. & pross. in household industry	Maf. & pross. other than household industry	Constru-ction	Total Secondary Sector	Trade & Commerce	Transport, storage & commun-ication	Other Services	Total Tertiary Sector
Uttarkashi	77.55	1.32	2.81	**81.68**	0.71	0.80	2.41	**3.92**	2.62	0.60	11.18	**14.40**
Chamoli	73.10	0.84	1.60	**75.54**	1.16	1.15	2.61	**4.92**	3.16	1.08	15.30	**19.54**
Tehri	77.93	1.01	1.32	**80.26**	0.30	1.20	4.20	**5.70**	2.82	1.15	10.07	**14.04**
Dehradun	22.43	9.50	3.58	**35.51**	0.86	11.34	4.78	**16.98**	11.71	4.45	31.35	**47.51**
Pauri	62.40	1.80	2.48	**66.68**	0.51	2.08	2.61	**5.20**	4.31	1.90	21.91	**28.12**
Pithoragarh	73.46	0.77	1.34	**75.57**	1.62	0.82	1.74	**4.18**	3.51	0.99	15.74	**20.25**
Almora	76.49	0.93	1.67	**79.09**	0.71	0.89	1.74	**3.34**	3.28	1.04	13.25	**17.57**
Nainital	41.15	18.49	3.23	**62.87**	0.94	7.55	2.87	**11.36**	8.34	3.29	14.14	**25.77**
Uttarakhand	**58.13**	**6.40**	**2.40**	66.93	**0.86**	**4.21**	**2.93**	8.00	**5.78**	**2.16**	**17.13**	25.07
India	**38.72**	**26.09**	**2.72**	67.53	**2.38**	**7.65**	**1.94**	11.97	**7.45**	**2.80**	**10.25**	20.50

Source: Anon, 1991a.

(33.79%) average (4.8). Similarly the proportion of main workers varies from 31.9% in Pauri to 48% in Uttarkashi. One important feature of the Uttarakhand is the presence of a substantial high proportion of female workers in workforce but it does not indicate the better life of females. It only shows their servitude to the hard economic life of their habitat. Females in general are engaged in low productive activities in the primary sector.

The work participation rate among females is higher (25.62%) in Uttarakhand compared to the country (15.79%). Likewise the marginal workers among female population are also registered higher (9.73%) as compared to the country (6.26%) as a whole. The proportion of main workers among females is registered considerable lower in the districts of Nainital (11.96%) and Dehradun (10.80%). Remaining districts of Uttarakhand, the female work participation rate as main workers is registered highest 44.99% in Uttarkashi while it is 38.72 in Almora, 36.50% in Pithoragarh, 39.83% in Chamoli, 36.38% in Tehri and 23.66% in Pauri (Table 4.8). About 58.13% of the total main workers in the region are engaged in cultivation in comparison to 38.72% of the country. In the two semi-hill districts of Nainital and Dehradun, where the land is plain and soil is fertile and modern techniques of cultivation are in practice, the percentage of workers in total populaton is lower than those of purely hill districts where topography is undulating and traditional methods of cultivation are in practice, as a result, agriculture in the hills is highly labour-intensive, reflects the high percentage of workers in the cultivation. The proportion of agricultural labourers to the total main workers in the region is 6.4% as against 26.9% in the country. Except Nainital and Dehradun districts, the percentage of agricultural labourers in the total workforce is almost negligible (Table 4.8). The proportion of main workers engaged in household industry is 0.86% as compared to 2.38% in country.

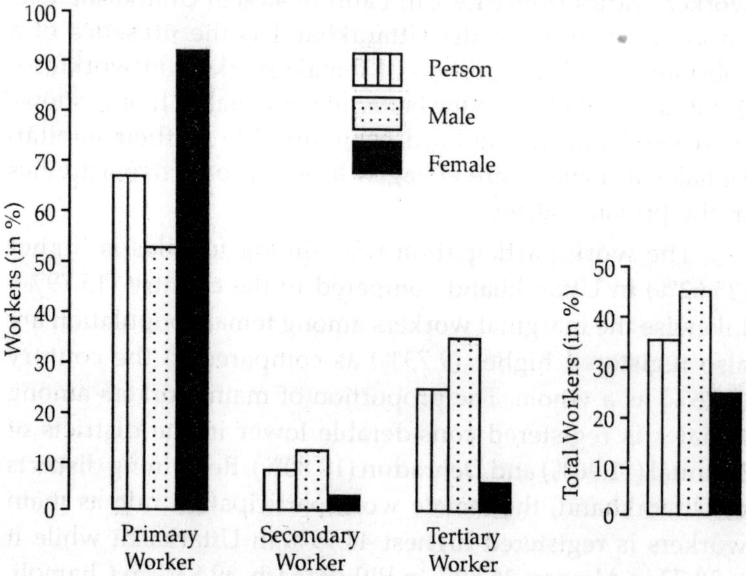

Fig. 4.7. Labour-Force Participation in Uttarakhand, 1991.

The occupational classification of female workers in the region indicates that about 93.16%, 1.52% and 5.32% of them are engaged in primary sector (cultivation, agricultural labourers, quarrying, mining etc.), secondary sector (household industries, construction etc.) and tertiary sector (trade, commerce, transport and other services), respectively. Table 4.9 shows the sector wise overall male-female labourforce participation in the region.

4.1.7 Reserved Category Population

According to the 1991 census, about 16.7% of the population belonged to Scheduled Caste and 3.5% to Scheduled Tribes. However, castewise census has not been done since 1931. There is no authentic and reliable information about Other Backward Classes (*OBC*).

Table 4.9. Labour Force Participation in Uttarakhand, 1991

Occupation	*Persons*	*Male*	*Female*
Primary Sector*	66.93	53.16	93.16
Secondary sector*	8.00	11.40	1.52
Tertiary Sector*	25.07	35.44	5.32
Total workers **	36.36	46.61	25.62
Marginal Workers**	5.56	1.72	9.57
Non-Workers**	58.08	51.67	64.81

Source: Pant, 2000a
*Percentage to the total workers.
**Percentage to the total population.

(i) Scheduled Caste Population: About 16.7% of the population in Uttarakhand belongs to Scheduled Castes – the Uttarkashi district having maximum (22.78%) and Dehradun district the minimum (13.40%). The sex ratio in the Scheduled Caste population is 937 females/1000 males. In 1981, 24.87% of the Scheduled Caste population were literates, compared 39.34% literacy of the total population. Of these, 38.20% are males and 10.47% females. The highest (20%) female literacy was registered in the Dehradun district followed by the Pauri district having 13% only. Nearly 37.88% Scheduled Caste population is considered as main workers more than 70% being engaged in the primary sector (agriculture) (Table 4.10).

(ii) **Scheduled Tribe Population:** About 3.54% of the Uttarakhand population belongs to the Scheduled Tribes, the highest 8.2% being in the Dehradun district, and 5.84% in the Nainital district. The tribal include Tharu, Buksha, Bhotia, Raji, and Jaunsari people. Tharus and Bukshas are confined to Tarai-Bhabar belt of Nainital district, while the Bhotia live in northern Pithoragarh and Chamoli districts and the Jaunsaris are confined to the Chakrata tehsil in the Dehradun district. The average literacy among the Scheduled Tribe is 23.56% and the sex ratio is 930 females/1000 males. The highest 1056 females

Table 4.10. Demographic Characteristics of Scheduled Castes Population in Uttarakhand, 1991

District/ Region	*Total (T) Rural (R) Urban (U)*	*Total Population*	*% of Scheduled Castes population to total population*	*Density (Persons per km²)*	*Sex Ratio (Females per 1000 Males)*	*Literacy (1981) (%)*			*% of Main Workers (1981)*
						Person	*Male*	*Female*	
1	2	3	4	5	6	7	8	9	10
	T	54,594	22.78	7	944	15.46	27.45	3.01	54.94
Uttarkashi	R	52,355	23.54	6	950	14.74	26.63	2.57	55.42
	U	2,239	12.97	132	806	34.38	45.67	17.43	42.08
	T	79,572	17.49	9	977	23.88	40.63	6.55	46.06
Chamoli	R	72,837	17.58	8	997	22.26	38.94	5.45	46.57
	U	6,735	16.61	102	784	43.16	57.99	22.32	40.06
	T	82,384	14.20	19	981	15.21	27.85	2.53	46.92
Tehri	R	79,013	14.44	18	993	14.55	27.11	2.03	47.24
	U	3,371	10.25	69	739	37.70	50.01	21.82	37.70
	T	1,37,464	13.40	45	851	32.25	42.27	20.04	33.67
Dehradun	R	77,287	15.15	26	846	26.88	37.12	14.36	36.40
	U	60,177	11.67	743	858	38.65	48.40	26.78	30.42

	T	92,261	13.52	17	1013	29.03	45.61	13.00	28.12
Pauri	R	83,640	13.91	16	1037	27.48	44.38	11.62	38.81
	U	8,621	10.62	127	814	43.44	55.30	28.12	28.12
	T	1,84,237	22.02	34	1018	25.32	40.43	10.41	32.70
Almora	R	1,75,702	22.44	32	1027	24.18	39.19	9.11	32.71
	U	8,535	15.95	275	846	55.94	65.45	43.80	32.48
	T	2,43,314	15.80	36	866	24.47	34.97	11.85	34.43
Nainital	R	1,86,858	18.02	28	872	22.97	34.12	9.56	35.71
	U	56,456	11.22	565	846	30.33	38.33	20.77	29.42
	T	1,15,832	20.45	13	956	25.53	41.51	8.85	38.25
Pithoragarh	R	1,09,234	20.83	12	964	24.67	40.69	8.05	38.60
	U	6,598	15.67	314	840	45.15	58.52	28.73	30.23
	T	**9,89,658**	**16.70**	**19**	**937**	**24.87**	**38.20**	**10.47**	**37.88**
Uttarakhand	**R**	**8,36,926**	**18.04**	**16**	**955**	**22.82**	**36.67**	**8.28**	**39.00**
	U	**1,52,732**	**11.88**	**253**	**843**	**37.43**	**47.22**	**25.39**	**30.80**

Source: Anon, 1981a, 1991a and Pant, 1996a.

Table 4.11. Demographic Characteristics of Scheduled Tribe Population in Uttarakhand, 1991

District/ Region	*Total (T) Rural (R) Urban (U)*	*Total Population*	*% of Scheduled Tribes population to total population*	*Density (Persons per km²)*	*Sex Ratio (Females per 1000 Males)*	*Literacy (1981) (%)*			*% of Main Workers (1981)*
						Person	*Male*	*Female*	
1	2	3	4	5	6	7	8	9	10
	T	2300	0.96	0.29	909	40.84	57.53	22.01	42.98
Uttarkashi	R	2240	1.01	0.28	908	40.28	57.04	21.58	43.00
	U	60	0.35	3.53	935	59.61	71.88	40.00	42.31
	T	10073	2.26	1.12	1062	45.88	63.11	29.43	36.84
Chamoli	R	7939	1.92	0.87	1113	40.03	58.11	23.56	36.43
	U	2334	5.76	35.36	907	60.79	74.81	45.70	37.89
	T	615	0.11	0.14	1312	57.35	63.27	42.11	45.59
Tehri	R	548	0.10	0.13	1491	52.46	59.09	35.29	45.90
	U	67	0.20	1.40	456	100.00	100.00	100.00	42.86
	T	84046	8.20	27.23	889	18.64	29.36	60.08	47.06
Dehradun	R	81005	15.88	26.95	898	18.13	28.78	5.72	47.68
	U	3071	0.60	37.91	684	61.31	67.43	48.45	41.24

	T	1502	0.22	0.28	744	26.16	40.22	6.55	41.20
Pauri	R	1358	0.23	0.25	784	19.35	32.55	2.35	38.22
	U	144	0.18	2.12	440	80.99	87.64	62.50	65.29
	T	2739	0.33	0.51	949	46.57	61.39	31.55	39.86
Almora	R	2044	0.26	0.38	1018	44.55	60.76	27.87	40.53
	U	695	1.30	22.42	773	60.36	65.91	55.24	35.27
	T	90020	5.84	13.25	944	19.04	31.59	6.12	28.53
Nainital	R	88061	8.49	13.16	947	18.71	31.15	5.95	28.58
	U	1959	0.39	19.59	814	48.61	64.96	25.07	23.82
	T	18313	3.23	2.07	995	47.62	62.41	32.51	36.99
Pithoragarh	R	15140	2.89	1.71	982	44.66	59.96	29.07	37.69
	U	3173	7.53	151.09	1056	68.94	79.87	57.57	31.96
	T	**209838**	**3.54**	**4.10**	**930**	**23.56**	**35.64**	**10.43**	**38.10**
Uttarakhand	**R**	**198335**	**4.27**	**3.91**	**935**	**22.03**	**34.06**	**9.03**	**38.21**
	U	**11503**	**0.89**	**26.57**	**843**	**62.27**	**73.79**	**48.28**	**32.52**

Source: Anon, 1981a, 1991a and Pant, 1996a.

per 1000 males ratio is seen in the Pithoragarh district. The main working population is 38% - the highest 47.6% being in the Dehradun district and the minimum 28.53% in the Nainital district (Table 4.11).

4.1.8 Ex-Service Men

There are over 30,000 men serving in the armed forces alone, and about 3,03,713 (6.3% of the population) experienced, well trained and disciplined ex-service men (Table 4.12) are available for participation in manifold meaningful programmes of development of the region (Valdiya, 1996). Maximum 65,716 ex-servicemen reside in Pithoragarh district and minimum 5000 are in Uttarkashi. Pauri and Almora districts having almost equal about 48 thousand ex-service men (Table 4.12).

Table 4.12. Ex-Servicemen of Uttarakhand, 1989–90

District/Region	*Population (1981)*	*No. of Ex-Servicemen*
Uttarakashi	1,91,000	5,000
Chamoli	3,64,000	31,000
Tehri	4,98,000	19,978
Dehradun	7,62,000	25,500
Pauri	6,40,000	48,232
Pithoragarh	4,89,000	65,716
Almora	7,57,000	48,194
Nainital	11,37,000	24,093
Uttarakhand	48,38,000	3,03,713

Source: Valdiya, 1996.

4.2 Fairs and Festivals

It is well known fact that Uttarakhand is a meeting place for various cultural groups which were came down from the Central Asia in the north and the Gangetic plain in the south. Its western and eastern limits are respectively demarcated by the Himachal Pradesh and Nepal. Consequently one can see the creative influence of surroundings on the Uttarakhand region. There are number of fairs celebrated by the

Uttarakhand people among them Jauljibi, Thal, Uttarayani, Janmastami, Shivratri, Nandadevi, Syalde Bikhoti, Somnath (Masi), Kedar, Binsar, Devidhura, Jageshwar, Punyagiri, Hatkalika, Kote ki mai, Gauchar, Chandrabadani, Ramnavami, Chaitra Astami, (Deghat & Kalinka), Mostamanu, Nandadevi Rajjat, Chhiplajat, Hill jatra, Kandali, Chamu Jat are important one.

The people of Uttarakhand celebrate all the major Indian festivals like Holi, Navratri, Diwali, Muharram, Barawafat, Sha-be-raat, Id-ul-fitar, Id-ul-zuha, Easter, Christmas, Baisakhi, Gurunanak Jayanit. Maker Sankranti, Basant Panchami, Harela, Bhitauli, Phool Dei, Olgia or Ghee Sankranti, Bat Savitri, Ganga Dushera, Rakshabandhan, Ghuiya Ekadashi, Krishna Janmastami, Shivratri, Nandastami, Saton Aathon, Ramnavami, Nag Panchami are some of the majors festivals of Uttarakhand. The Uttarakhandi ritual and food preparations have their own uniqueness. These preparations are related with every aspects of life from birth to death.

4.3 Landuse and Allied Sectors

The total reporting area of Uttarakhand is recorded 53,72,625 hectares during 1989-90. The landuse statistics showed that out of the total reported area, 64% of land is under forests, 5.62% culturable waste land, 0.14% under current fallow, 1.13% other fallows, 5.30% not suitable for cultivation, 2.44% land other than cultivation, 3.94% considered as permanent pastures and grazing land, 3.81% under trees, bushes, gardens, excluding cultivation and 13.62% net cultivated area during 1989-90 (Table 4.13 and Figure 4.8).

Cropping pattern denotes to the proportion of the area given to different crops in a particular crop season. Table 4.14 shows the districtwise area under various crops in Rabi and Kharif seasons. Paddy and madua are two major crops in Kharif foodgrain while wheat and barely are in Rabi foodgrains. About 38.62% of the net sown area is devoted to paddy while 53.45% area under wheat crop. Remaining corn and barely are the other principal crops in the region.

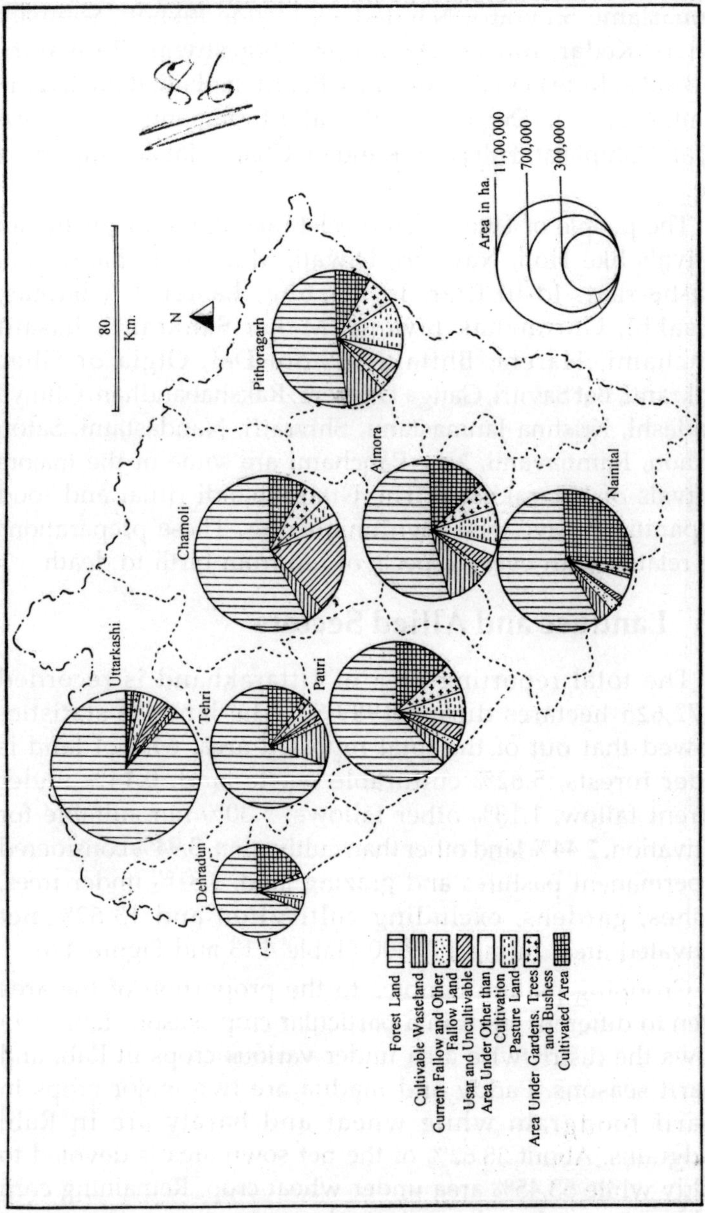

Fig. 4.8. Major Landuse in Uttarakhand, 1989–90.

Table 4.13. Major Landuse in Uttarakhand, 1989-1990

Particulars	*Uttarkashi*	*Pauri*	*Chamoli*	*Tehri*	*Dehradun*	*Almora*	*Nainital*	*Pithoragarh*	*Uttarakhand*
Reported Area (ha)	**8,01,619**	**7,57,994**	**8,55,206**	**5,74,543**	**3,14,899**	**7,26,881**	**7,04,344**	**6,37,139**	**53,72,625**
Forest	88.60	59.32	62.55	69.13	69.62	53.95	57.52	51.84	**64.00**
Cultivable waste land	1.08	5.67	3.78	12.72	3.56	7.75	3.98	7.72	**5.62**
Current fallow	0.01	0.02	0.01	0.01	0.69	0.08	0.48	0.16	**0.14**
Other fallow	0.46	2.28	0.18	1.47	1.29	1.01	0.96	1.80	**1.13**
Usar and not suitable for cultivation	2.39	4.37	18.71	2.13	0.54	4.15	0.65	3.71	**5.30**
Area under other uses excluding cultivation	0.82	2.23	2.05	1.92	5.37	2.25	4.52	2.17	**2.44**
Permanent pasture and other grazing lands	1.66	5.53	2.48	0.50	0.01	7.82	0.16	11.67	**3.94**
Area under trees, bushes, gardens excluding cultivated area	0.91	7.86	4.01	–	1.37	5.99	2.21	6.32	**3.81**
Net cultivated area	4.07	12.72	6.23	12.12	17.55	17.00	29.52	14.61	**13.62**
(a) Kharif cropped area*	100.00	97.38	91.45	100.00	88.16	99.88	93.93	94.34	**95.67**
(b) Rabi cropped area*	52.56	55.29	50.88	61.35	70.40	66.70	71.57	73.39	**65.41**
(c) Jaid cropped area*	–	–	–	–	4.26	–	3.36	–	**1.28**
(d) Area under sugarcane*	–	–	–	–	–	–	0.05	–	**0.02**
(e) Gross cropped area*	152.56	152.67	142.33	161.35	162.82	166.58	168.91	167.73	**162.38**

Source: Anon, 1992.
* % of net cultivated area

Table 4.14. Area Under Kharif and Rabi Crops, 1989-1990

Crops	*Uttarkashi*	*Chamoli*	*Tehri*	*Dehradun*	*Pauri*	*Pithoragarh*	*Almora*	*Nainital*	*Uttarakhand*
Kharif crops (% of Kharif cropped area)									
Paddy	34.85	37.71	24.01	24.63	26.54	49.76	33.45	56.46	38.62
Corn	2.05	1.05	2.32	24.59	2.38	5.64	2.18	3.99	4.67
Madua (Ragi)	22.44	30.15	27.83	8.08	34.90	27.95	40.14	3.01	21.98
Sawan (Jhungora)	12.07	8.26	33.42	3.63	24.22	5.60	17.47	0.62	11.57
Urd	1.85	0.61	2.27	1.77	3.93	1.04	1.14	0.62	1.38
Others	26.74	22.22	10.15	37.30	8.03	10.01	5.62	35.66	21.78
Total	**100.00**	**100.00**	**100.00**	**100.00**	**100.00**	**100.00**	**100.00**	**100.00**	**100.00**
Rabi Crop: (% of Rabi cropped area)									
Wheat	44.46	45.07	51.30	54.83	44.26	75.69	84.34	82.48	53.45
Barley	1.48	3.70	6.57	4.37	8.49	11.88	8.79	0.94	4.70
Lentil	01.19	0.13	1.35	2.08	0.75	7.67	3.20	3.17	02.17
Gram	0.03	–	0.02	0.43	0.07	0.07	0.11	0.95	0.26
Mater	0.19	0.04	0.15	0.45	0.02	0.09	0.05	0.59	0.20
Arhar (Tur)	0.39	0.19	0.86	0.13	0.50	0.01	0.01	0.17	0.23
Others	52.26	50.87	39.75	37.71	45.91	4.59	3.50	11.70	38.99
Total	**100.00**	**100.00**	**100.00**	**100.00**	**100.00**	**100.00**	**100.00**	**100.00**	**100.00**

Source: Anon, 1992 and Pant, 1998.

Table 4.15 indicates the district wise extent of irrigation during 1990-91 in the Uttarakhand Himalaya. It shows 34.91% of net sown area is irrigated. The figures related to irrigated areas of district Nainital and Dehradun are separated from the irrigated areas of rest of the hill districts, it is found that the proportion of irrigated area varies from 5.37% in district Chamoli to 15.26% in Uttarakashi, whereas the proportion of irrigated area is accounted 81.4% in district Nainital and 44.77% in Dehradun (Table 4.15).

Table 4.15. Irrigated Area in Uttarakhand, 1990-91

Districts/Region	*Area*	
	(ha)	*(% of net area sown)*
Uttarkashi	4,443	15.26
Chamoli	2,492	5.37
Tehri	10,024	13.90
Deharadun	22,444	44.77
Pauri	8,092	8.88
Almora	12,925	12.20
Nainital	1,67,676	81.40
Pithoragarh	5,524	8.08
Uttarakhand	**2,33,610**	**34.91**

Source: Anon, 1993.

According to Government Statistics for 1985-86, the total number of operational holdings in the Uttarakhand is 7.54 lakhs with an area of 7.1 lakhs ha. The average land holding size of the region is 0.94 ha which is more than the U.P. (0.93 ha). Districtwise land holding size varies from 0.54 ha. in Pithoragarh to 1.67 ha in Nainital district. Approximately 71% of the holding with 28.1% total cultivated of area are marginal holding i.e. below 1 ha. Below 2 ha holdings constitute about 88% of the operational holdings with 53.1% of the total cultivated area. The number of land holding size between 4 ha to 10 ha constitute about 3.0% of the total holdings in the region while the percentage of holdings which are above 10 ha are nearly 0.2%. The study reflects that small and marginal

Table 4.16. Number and Area of Operational Holdings in Uttarakhand, 1991-92

(% of Total)

District/ Region	Marginal (Below 1 ha)		Small (1-2 ha)		Semi Medium (2-4 ha)		Medium (4-10 ha)		Large (>10 ha)		Total	
	No.	Area	No.	Area	No.	Area	No.	Area	No.	Area	No.	Area
Uttarkashi	64.8	21.0	19.4	27.8	12.8	35.3	2.9	15.2	0.1	8.7	34,984	34,309
Chamoli	69.8	27.7	18.8	30.2	9.3	28.1	2.0	12.1	0.1	1.9	52,956	46,218
Tehri	69.3	30.5	21.1	35.2	8.4	26.3	1.2	7.5	*	0.5	88,547	74,109
Dehradun	76.9	37.8	12.6	21.4	7.8	22.0	2.5	13.8	0.2	5.0	69,750	67,496
Pauri	56.5	15.7	22.6	24.7	15.1	32.2	5.4	22.8	0.4	4.6	91,683	1,17,566
Almora	80.9	47.7	14.6	31.2	4.1	17.2	0.4	3.5	*	0.4	1,78,951	1,11,078
Pithoragarh	83.6	48.2	12.1	28.2	3.8	17.6	0.5	5.2	*	0.8	1,21,018	65,905
Nainital	55.4	14.6	18.3	16.0	17.2	29.0	8.1	27.9	1.0	12.5	1,16,609	1,94,291
Uttarakhand	**71.2**	**28.1**	**16.8**	**25.0**	**9.0**	**25.9**	**2.8**	**16.0**	**0.2**	**5.0**	**7,54,498**	**7,10,972**

Source: Joshi *et al.* 1999.*= Negligible

holdings are largest in number in the region (Table 4.16). On an average only 0.09 ha land goes to the per head share of the cultivated land in the region. Table 4.17 shows the decreasing trend of per capita agricultural land in the region since 1848 to 2001. The population pressure on cultivated, forest, and pasture lands is considerably high (Pant, 1992a).

Table 4.17. Per Capita Cultivated Land in Uttarakhand Since, 1848

Year	*Specified Region*	*Per Capita Land (in ha)*	*Source*
1848	Kumaun	1.6	Batten, 1848
1874	Kumaun	0.47	Backett, 1874
1896	Garhwal	0.65	Pauw, 1896
1865	Dehradun	0.55	Baker, 1886
1885	Himalaya West	0.55	Baker, 1886
1921	Himalaya West	0.68	Census, 1921
1931	Himalaya West	0.63	Census, 1931
1941	Himalaya West	0.55	Census, 1941
1951	Himalaya West	0.41	Census, 1951
1991	Kumaun	0.14	Census, 1991
1991	Uttarakhand	0.12	Census, 1991
2001	Uttarakhand	0.09	Census, 2001

Source: Pant, 1992b and Anon, 2001.

The environment of the region is optimum for growing the sub-tropical and temperate fruits. Out of total 1,60,353 ha reported area under fruits, 31.90% area covers by apple trees followed by citrus fruits contain 11.57% area. Litchi and Mango encompasses an area of 10.6% and 10.88% of total area under fruits trees. Maximum 47.25% and 40.9% of the total area is under apple in Uttarkashi and Nainital district respectively (Pant, 1995a).

During 1987-88 about 37,783 ha area under vegetables in the region. Dehradun and Nainital districts which have more urban population and ample irrigated area as compared to other purely hilly districts. Potato cultivation is spread all over the region because of its number of varieties and high acclimatization capacity in different elevation. Notwithstandingly only 13,038 ha area is under potato cultivation. Every type of root and leafy vegetables including mushroom, cabbage, pumpkin, onion, ladies finger, capsicum, pea, tomato, cauliflower, frenchbean, spinach, potato, redish, brinjal, etc. are grown in the region.

Floriculture is also another great avenue for the development because the environmental condition of the region is very conductive to grow various types of flowers including glaidoli, marigold, jasmine, rose, etc.

The tea plantation was started in 1830 in Uttarakhand and unfortunately now it is observed that a number of uncared old tea garden in the region are in the process of being removed by the private owners. However, few schemes for new plantation and establishment of private garden (joint enterprenureship of land owner and Govt.) are launching in recent decade. An estimation that there are 12,000 ha of land in Uttarakhand suitable for tea gardening and the potential of generating Rs. 150 crores and providing employment to 30,000 persons. The productivity of the plantation is merely 1000 kg/ha (Ramit Joshi, per. Com.). The Uttarakhand Himalaya has lot of scope for mushroom cultivation. Presently few centers are established for its cultivation.

In 1982, there are 39,41,641 animals in Uttarakhand, of which 49.92% of cows, 18.9% of baffaloes, 10.4% of sheep. 21.3% of goats, 0.34% of horses and 0.5% of porks. It is observed that the quality of livestock population is very low, consequently the byproducts of the animals are also low. The milk production in Uttarakhand in the year 1986-87 was 50,100 tons largely from the milch animals of Tarai-Bhabar and dun belts (Dhar & Gupta, 1992).

4.4 Food Production and Nutrition Availability

Paddy (rice), wheat, corn, madua, sawan (Jhungra), barley, urd, peas, arhar, lentil, moong are the important and reported kharif and rabi foodgrains in Uttarakhand. Study shows the net available foodgrains, vegetables (potato and onion), pulses, cooking oil and per capita availability of these items in Uttarakhand Himalaya (Pant, 1998) excluding the other edible items on an average the cereal production in the area is in excess. Hence, it is a common phenomenon that the people purchase the other edible items in lie of cereals. The marginal and small landholders also purchase the foodgrains from the other sources, i.e., market and big landholders.

With the help of food composition tables which are prepared by the experts of the Indian council of Medical Research Hyderabad, the total agricultural produce has been converted into various important nutrients, viz. energy, protein, fat, carbohydrates, calcium, iron, carotene, riboflavin, and niacin. Considering the daily minimum requirement of energy is about 2500 kcal per capita particularly for this region in which nearly 70% of the total energy is gained from the available cereals, pulses, onion, and potato. Remaining 30% energy is gained from the fruits, flesh, milk, sugar, other root and leafy vegetables, cooking oil and spices which are not considered here due to the paucity of the reliable data of these items. However, an attempt has been made to examine the availability of cereals are 484.67 grams, pulses 7.43, edible oil 1.63, potato 80.31 and onion is 5.47 grams in the region. With these items the per capita per day energy intake derives 1760.17 kcal, protein 26.81 grams, fat 9.17 grams, carbohydrates 372.5 grams, calcium 384.49 mg, iron 20.66 μg, carotene 181.84 mg, thiamine 1.95 mg, riboflavin 0.8 mg, and 21.24 mg niacin in the region (Pant, 1998). It is also worth to mention that there are some prominent deficiency diseases prevailing in the various segments of the society. This is mainly because of the ignorance, illiteracy and the poverty (Pant, 1998).

4.5 State of Infrastuctural Development

A number of institutions which provide maximum facilities to its inhabitants are the appropriate indicators to understand the socio-economic status of the region. Keeping in mind the ratio between the number of institutions established in the region and population Uttarakhand does not present a picture to undeveloped region but if undulating ground would be consider the real picture of the region would be clear. Due to difficult topography and lack of transport means one can not get benefit from these available institutions. The basic infrastructural indicators of development in Uttarakhand can be seen in table 4.18.

Generally speaking, the physical environmental conditions of Uttarakhand are quite good for the helath point of view. But there are many negative casues which adversely affect their health. Inaccessibility, rough terrain, poor nutrition, unsafe water supply, poor sanitation and hygiene, tremendous pressure of work on women folk etc. have given rise to incidence of asthma, bronchitis, tuberculosis, eye diseases, stomach worms, infections, disease of malnutrition, abdominal disorders, stone formation etc. As already mentioned that the access to medical and health centers is quite restricted. The shortage of medical personals is endemic. There is an urgent need of special health planning due to difficult geographical conditions in the region. Table 4.18 gives a summary of some of the important medical and health facilities available in Uttarakhand. From the accessibility point of view about 56.7% of the villages in the hill district are located at distance exceeding five km from the nearest Allopathic Hospital/Dispensary/PHCs, 16.9% are located at distance varying from three to five km. Similarly, 43.2% of the villages are located at distance exceeding five km from the nearest Maternity and Child Welfare Center or sub-Center (Dhar, 1996). The overall development of the region is quite poor as can be seem from table 4.20. Table shows that the fully hill districts are least developed even the index of development has registered negative growth.

Table 4.18. Basic Infrastructural Indicator of Development in Uttarakhand

Indicators (Most relate to 1991-92)	*Uttarakhand*
1. Mettaled Road per 1000 km^2 of area (km)	227
2. No. of Schools / 100,000 people	
• Primary	144
• Senior Basic	30
• Higher Secondary	19
3. Medical Facilities / 100,000 people	
• Allopathic Hospitals / Dispensaries	12.41
• Beds in Allopathic Hospitals / Dispensaries	121.84
• Primary Health Centres	3.6
• Sub-Centres / Maternity Service Centres	27.49
4. Electricity	
• Per Capita Consumption	217.10
• % Villages Electrified	73.53
5. Communication (Per 100,000 people)	
• Post Office	42.7
• Telephone Connection	395
• Telegraph Offices	11.6
6. Technical Education / 100,000 people	
• Industrial Training Institute (ITI)	1.06
• Polytechnics	0.29
7. No. of Bank Branches, per 1,00,000 people	11.5

Source: Papola, 2000.

Table 4.19. Medical and Health facilities Available in Uttarakhand at the Beginning of the Eighth Plan

	Item	*Units*
	Hospitals (Allopathic)	
(i)	Rural	50
(ii)	Urban	16
	Dispensaries (Allopathic)	
(i)	Urban	6
(ii)	Rural	331
	Hospital Beds	
(i)	Urban	2137
(ii)	Rural	3098
	Health Centres	
(i)	Sub Centres	1432
(ii)	Primary Health Centres	247
(iii)	Communities Health Centres	19
	Hospital Bed – Population Ratio	1.868
	Doctor – Population Ratio	1.3543
•	Special Facilities (as on April 1st, 1992) Available in the Region	
	Pathology	33
	Radiology	17
	Orthopaedics	12
	Anaesthesiology	23
	Intensive Coronary Care Units	12
	Paediatrics	33
	Dentistry	38
	Emergency Services	10
	E.N.T.	12
	Blood Bank	2

Source: Dhar, 1996.

Table 4.20. Districtwise Level of Development of Uttarakhand

Particulars	*Almora*	*Chamoli*	*Dehradun*	*Pauri*	*Nainital*	*Pithoragarh*	*Tehri*	*Uttarakashi*
Relative Index of Development	46	38	142	51	132	55	40	47
% of Urbanisation	6.4	8.91	5.26	11.86	32.66	7.44	5.67	7.2
Level of Agricultural Development Value	– 0.38	– 0.64	– 1.10	– 0.62	– 0.87	– 0.45	– 0.52	– 0.38
Rank	296	330	364	329	47	308	318	294
Level of Development Manufacturing Value	– 1.17	– 1.06	0.70	– 1.16	0.16	– 1.34	– 1.7	– 1.43
Rank	337	321	89	335	145	353	366	358
Level of Development in Service Value	– 0.60	– 0.51	– 1.59	– 0.45	0.27	– 0.71	– 0.72	– 0.49
Rank	227	205	16	195	81	255	258	202
Level of Development in Industrialization Overall Value	– 0.65	– 0.66	0.54	– 0.65	0.44	– 0.76	– 0.86	– 0.65
Rank	317	323	63	318	79	342	351	319

Source: Bora, 2000

4.6 Accessibility

During the early 20th century, the region was completely traveled by on foot. Only some important towns such as Dehradun, Almora, Ranikhet, Mussoorie, Kotdwar, Lansdown, Kathgodam, Haldwani, Tanakpur and Pauri were accessible by motor vehicles. After the Chinese and Pak aggressions (1962, 1965 and 1971) in India after independence, the pace of development of transport network in the region has been accelerated and number of new roads have been constructed upto the interior places such as Narayan Ashram, Song, Munsyari, Pankhu, Manch, Tamli, Mandoli, Sonprayag, Ghuttu, Badiyargarh, Chauki, Budhakedar, Akhorhi, Sakari, Gangotri, Nagchulakhal, Thalisain, Bungidhar, Ghatgarh-Deghat, Betalghat, Patkot, Kunjakharak, Chopta, Malari, etc. (Fig. 4.9) in one hand while most of the remote village are still inaccessible by the motor vehicles. The roads in the region are mostly lying along the river valleys.

Pantnagar and Jollygrant are connected by airways with Delhi while Auli, Badrinath, Gauchar and Nainisaini are being connected with Dehradun, Pantnagar and Delhi by helicopter services. The foothill towns of Dehradun, Rishikesh, Kotdwar, Ramnagar, Kathgodam and Tanakpur are connected by the railways with Hardwar, Najimabad, Bareilly, Rampur and Pilibhit which are also well connected with Muradabad, Delhi, Lucknow and Agra.

Although the region is well connected with the town of plains by the metallic roads and railways. The north-eastern part is connected by the footpaths with Tibet and Nepal respectively. Western part is also connected by roads with Shimla, Chandigarh and Ambala. The length of moderable roads was about 13,532 km in 1987–88 –2,097 km in Almora district, 2,799 in Nainital, 1,188 in Pithoragarh, 803 in Uttarkashi, 2,202 in Pauri, 1192 in Chamoli, 1,353 in Tehri and 1,898 km in Dehradun district. However maximum villages of the region are well connected with one another by *kachcha* (Kharanja) paths.

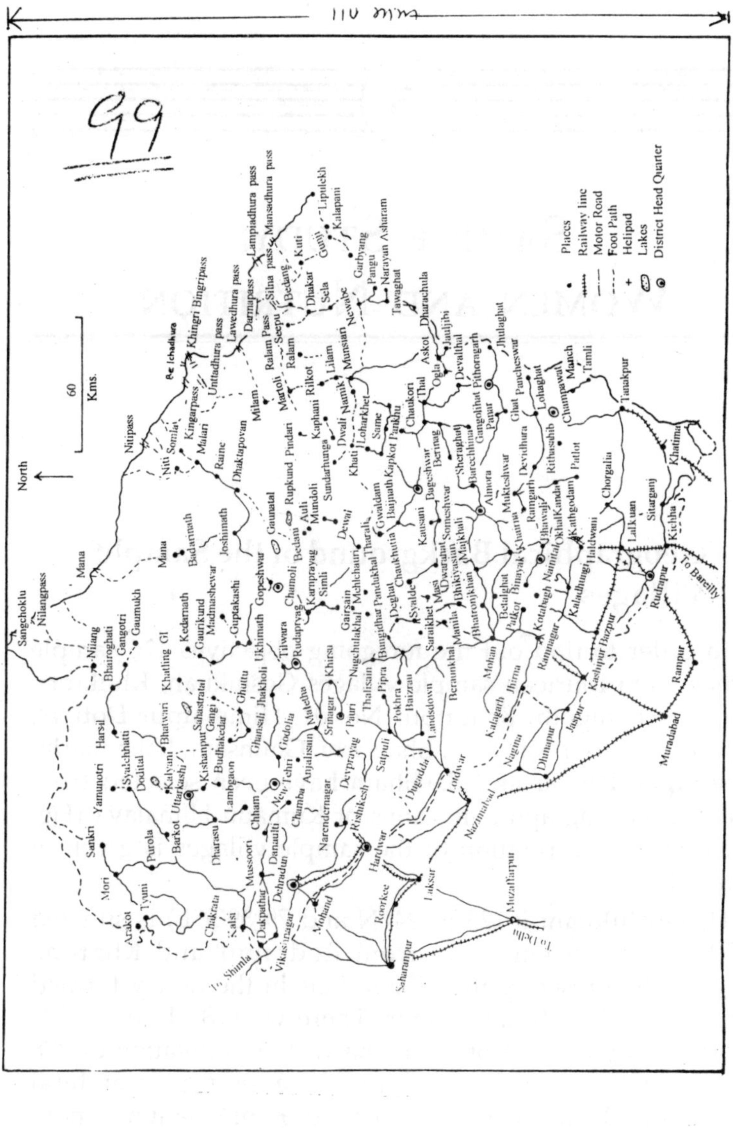

Fig. 4.9. Transport Network in Uttarakhand.

5

Sample Study: Women and Nutrition

5.1 Geographical Background of the Sample Villages

In order to find out the foregoing objectives 136 sample women from fourteen sample villages Goshikuan, Khukreta, Thari, Chchenigoth, Bharatpur No. 01, Himmatpur Dotiyal, Ramdatt, Haripur Kaliajala, Bhaisorhi, Ghunsera, Lakhanarhi, Chhetrapal, Pachar and Bachham have been selected from different physiographic divisions of Kumaun Himalaya (Fig. 5.1). General information of the sample villages is given in Table 5.1.

(1) Goshikuan: It (28°57′24″N and 79°59′5″E) is situated at 70 km and 5 km away from Rudrapur and Khatima respectively. Presently the village falls in the newly formed district of Udam Singh Nagar. There were 87 households encompassing an area of 177.66 ha with a population of 778 persons in 1999 which represents the eastern part of Tarai region. Total 10 women – 03 general (non-pregnant and non-lactating), 03 pregnant and 04 lactating category women have randomly been selected for the detailed study. The

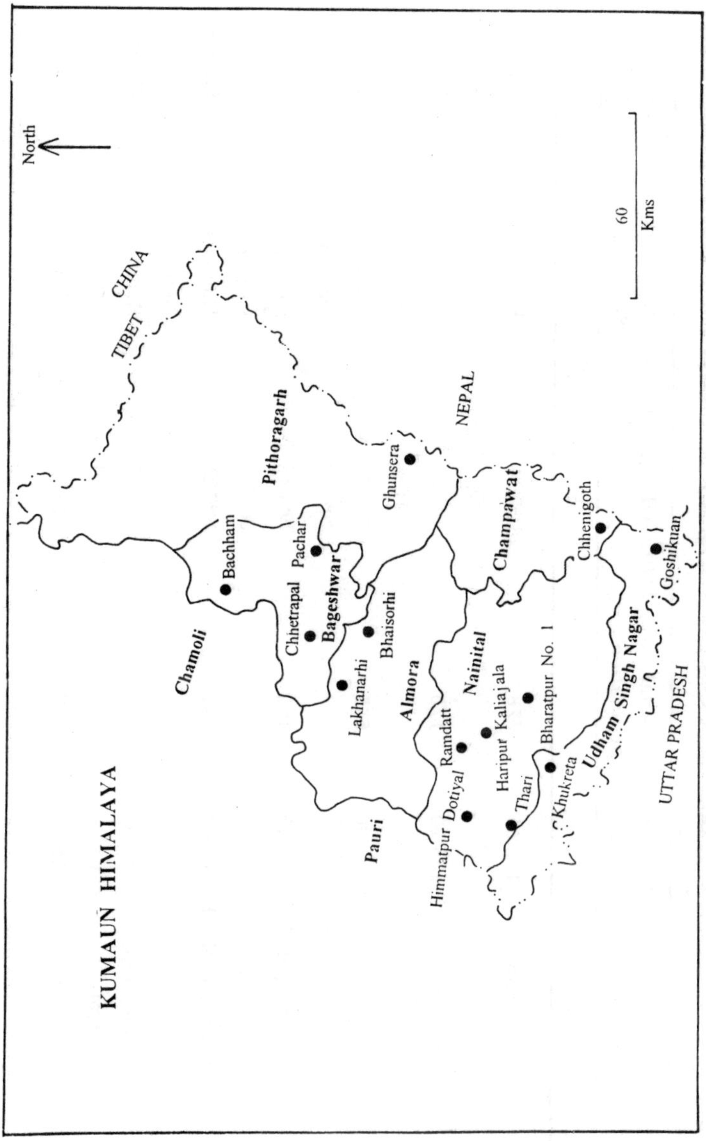

Fig. 5.1. Location of Sample Villages

Table 5.1. Sample Villages at a Glance

S. No.	*Name of the village*	*Total area (ha)*	*Total population*	*Latitude/Longitude*	*Development Block/District*	*Geographical Location*
1	2	3	4	5	6	7
1.	Goshikuan	177.66	778	28°57'24" N 79°59'5" E	Khatima/ U. S. Nagar	Tarai
2.	Khukreta	135.00	170	29°7'22" N 79°11'36" E	Bazpur/ U. S. Nagar	Tarai
3.	Thari	14.00	545	29°16'25" N 79°1'42" E	Ramnagar/ Nainital	Tarai
4.	Chchenigoth	21.45	192	29°4'16" N 80°7'10" E	Champawat/ Champawat	Bhabar
5.	Bharatpur No. 1	169.00	81	29°7'22" N 79°11'36" E	Haldwani/ Nainital	Bhabar
6.	Himmatpur Dotiyal	82.52	526	29°23'3" N 79°5'21" E	Ramnagar/ Nainital	Bhabar
7.	Ramdatt	25.09	167	29°24'29" N	Kotabagh/	Dun

8.	Haripur Kaliajala	42.49	159	29°21'16" N 79°19'20" E	Kotabagh/ Nainital	Dun
9.	Bhaisorhi	18.91	145	29°43' N 79°45' E	Takula/ Almora	Lesser Himalayan Mid slope
10.	Ghunsera	22.3	171	29°36'10" N 80°15'05" E	Pithoragarh/ Pithoragarh	Lesser Himalayan Mid slope
11.	Lakhanarhi	228.3	1849	29°46'41" N 79°38'54" E	Takula/ Almora	Lesser Himalayan Valley
12.	Chchetrapal	175.39	2083	29°54'24" N 79°39'29" E	Garur/ Bageshwar	Lesser Himalayan Valley
13.	Pachar	125.00	739	29°50'35" N 80°0'45" E	Kapkote/ Bagheswar	Lesser Himalayan Valley
14.	Bachcham	255.00	445	30°7'44" N 79°59'29" E	Kapkote/ Bageshwar	Close to Great Himalaya

environmental conditions of the region have already been discussed in Chapter III.

(2) Khukreta: Village Khukreta (29°7′22″ N and 79°11′36″E) 40 km and 11 km from Haldwani and Bazpur, respectively is situated in Bazpur development block. It encompasses an area of 135 ha with a population of 170 persons in 1999. It represents the central part of Tarai region, Similarly 10 sample women have been selected for the detailed study.

(3) Thari: Busksha (Scheduled Tribe) dominated village, Thari (29°16′25″N and 79°1′42″E) in Ramnagar development block is situated 20 km away from Ramnagar. It encompasses an area of 140 ha with total 545 persons in 1999. Ten Sample women – 03 from general, 04 from pregnant and 03 from lactating women have randomly been selected for the detailed study. It belongs to the western most part of the Tarai region.

(4) Chchenigoth: It (29°4′16″N and 80°7′10″E) is situated at about 8 km from Tanakpur. The village is completely surrounded by the dense forest. The revenue village encompasses an area of 21.45 ha with a population of 192 persons in 1999, which represents the eastern most part of Bhabar region. A total 10 sample women have been selected for the detailed study.

(5) Bharatpur No. 1: Village Bharatpur No. 1 (29°7′22″N and 79°11′36″E) 55 km and 10 km away from district headquarters Nainital and block headquarter Haldwani respectively. It encompasses an area of 169 ha and supports 81 persons in 1999. Out of total women, 06 sample i.e. two from each category have been selected for the detailed study.

(6) Himmatpur Dotiyal: Third and last sample village of Bhabar region, is the village Himmatpur Dotiyal (29°23′3″N and 79°5′21″E) in Ramnagar development block is situated at 74 km and 9 km away from Nainital and Ramnagar respectively. It encompasses an area of 82.52 ha and supports 526 persons in 1999. Out of total married women between the age of 19-45, 10 women have been selected for the sample study. The village is just below the Upper Siwalik range along Tanakpur-Kotdwar Kandi Road.

(7) Ramdatt: Ramdatt (29°24′29″N and 79°18′46″E) is situated at about 46 and one km away from district headquarter Nainital and block headquarter Kotabagh, respectively. The village lies in the Kotadun. It encompasses an area of 25.09 ha with a population of 167 persons in 1999 which represents the western part of Kotadun. Out of total married women between the age of 19-45 years, 10 women – 03 general, 03 pregnant and 04 lactating have been selected for the sample study.

(8) Haripur Kaliajala: Haripur Kaliajala (29°21′16″N and 79°19′20″E) 41 and 5 km away from Nainital and Kotábagh, respectively, is situated in Baur catchment of Kotadun. It encompasses an area of 42.49 ha with a total population of 159 persons in 1999. Out of total women, 10 women have randomly been selected for the detailed study.

(9) Bhaisorhi: Village Bhaisorhi (29°43′ N and 79°49′ E) is situated at 30 and 10 km away from district headquarters Almora and block headquarter Gananath (Takula) respectively. It encompasses an area of 18.91 ha with a total population of 145 persons in 1999. Out of total women, 10 women have been selected for the detailed study. The village is situated in mature terrain of the Lesser Himalaya.

(10) Ghunsera: Village Ghunsera (29°36′46″N and 80°11′10″E) is situated 5 km away from district headquarter of Pithoragarh. It encompasses of an area 22.3 ha with a total population of 275 persons in 1999. Out of total women, 10 women have randomly been selected for detailed study.

(11) Lakhanarhi: It (29°46′41″N and 79°38′ 54″E) is situated at about 40 km away from district headquarter Almora along Ranikhet – Gagas – Someshwar motor road. It encompasses an area of 65.2 ha with a population of 435 persons in 1999. Out of total women between the age of 19-45 year, 10 women –02 from general, 03 from pregnant and 05 from lactating women have randomly been selected for detailed study.

(12) Chhetrapal: Village Chhetrapal (29°54′24″N and 79°39′29″E) is situated in the terrace of Gomti river. It is 4 and 18 km away from block headquarter Garur and district headquarter Bageshwar respectively. It encompasses an area of 175.39 ha and supports 2083 persons in 2000. It is situated just 2 km away from the historical place of Baijnath. Similarly out of total women, 10 women between the age of 15-45 years have been randomly selected for detailed study.

(13) Pachar: It (29°50′35″N and 80°0′45″E) is situated about 55 km away both from district headquarter Bageshwar and block headquarter Kapkote respectively. It lies in Nakuri Patti of Pungar catchment. Out of total, 10 women –03 general, 04 pregnant and 03 lactating women have been selected for detailed study. It encompasses of an area 125 ha with a total population of 729 persons in 2000.

(14) Bachcham: Village Bachcham (30°7′44″N and 79°59′29″E) represents the villages situated in Higher Himalayan region. It is just near the Sundardhunga glacier and lies in Pindar catchment. It is situated about 20 km away from motor roadhead Song and 54 km and 30 km away from district headquarter Bageshwar and block headquarter Kapkote respectively. It lies in the way of famous Pindari and Sundardhunga glaciers. It encompasses an area of 250 ha and supports 250 persons in 2000. Out of total 10 women have been selected for detailed study (Tables 5.1 and 5.2).

5.2 Socio-Economic Status of the Sample Women

Before investigating the housing and environmental sanitation condition, hygiene pattern, dietary habits, amenities and food consumption, it is very important to know the socio- economic condition of the sample women in the villages which is very significant aspect to determine the nutrition and health status.

As has already been pointed out that for the purpose of this study some 136 women from 14 villages have been surveyed in six districts of Kumaun Himalaya.

Caste is a dominant feature within the village society. Several caste groups Brahmin, Chatriya (Rajput), Scheduled Castes (Silpkar-Craftsmen), Scheduled Tribe (Tharu and Buksha), Other Backward Classes (Goswami and Gujjar),

Rastogi (Kayastha), Nepali origin, Punjabi (Sikh) and Muslim are identified in the fourteen villages. These caste groups belong to Hindu, Muslim and Sikh religions. Three caste of Hindu – Brahmin, Chatriya and Silpkar are generally found in all villages but tribal villages and families such as Tharu, Buksha, Bhotia and Gujjar are situated in particular locations.

Table 5.2. Castewise Distribution of Sample Women

	Category of the Sample			
Caste	*General*	*Pregnant*	*Lactating*	*Total*
Brahmin	14 (35.90)	11 (25.00)	13 (24.53)	38 (27.94)
Chatriya (Rajput)	10 (25.65)	15 (34.09)	11 (20.75)	36 (26.47)
Scheduled Castes	02 (5.13)	04 (9.09)	11 (20.75)	17 (12.50)
Tharu (S.T.)	02 (5.13)	02 (4.55)	01 (1.89)	05 (3.68)
Buksha (S.T.)	03 (7.69)	03 (6.82)	03 (5.67)	09 (6.62)
Other Backward Classes	03 (7.69)	03 (6.82)	08 (15.09)	14 (10.29)
Sikh	03 (7.69)	03 (6.82)	06 (11.32)	12 (3.82)
Muslim	01 (2.56)	02 (4.55)	–	03 (2.21)
Rastogi (Kayastha)	01 (2.56)	01 (2.26)	–	02 (1.47)
Total	**39 (28.68) (100)**	**44 (32.35) (100)**	**53 (38.97) (100)**	**136 (100) (100)**

Source: Field Survey, 1999-2000.

Note: Figures shown in parenthesis refer to percentage of the total sample women.

Out of total 136 sample – 38 (27.94%) sample women are Brahmin, 36 (26.47%) Chatriya, 17 (12.5%) Scheduled Castes, 14 (10.30%) Scheduled Tribe, (09(6.62%) Buksha and 05 (3.68%) Tharu), 12 (8.82%) Punjabi, 02 (1.47%) Rastogi, 14 (10.29%).

Other Backward Classes and 03 (2.21%) are Muslims (Table 5.2). Out of total 136 sample women 39 (28.68%) sample women are non-pregnant non-lactating (in further details it is mentioned as general category) 44 (32.35%) pregnant and 53 (38.97%) are lactating women.

Keeping in mind the objectives of the study total sample women have been categorised into three age groups below 18 years, 19-45 years and 46-60 years. Data regarding the distribution of sample women according to age groups is presented in table 5.3, which indicates that only 2.2% women were less than 18 years of age and about 8% were in age group 46-60 years. Maximum sample about 90% were belong to the workforce age group between the age of 19 to 45 years. The table indicates that still the marriage age of the girls prevails below 18 years in the rural areas as against the Marriage Act. Even among them (below 18 years age), one woman was found pregnant in the village Chchetrapal and two women were lactating category respectively in Haripur Kaliajala and Khukreta villages. Between the age of 46 to 60 years only one woman was found pregnant during the survey in village Chchenigoth except this all 10 sample in this group (46-60 years) were in general category.

Table 5.3. Age Structure of the Sample

Age Group (in Years)	*Category of the Sample*			*Total*
	General	*Pregnant*	*Lactating*	
Below 18	–	01 (2.27)	02 (3.77)	03 (2.21)
19-45	29 (74.36)	42 (95.46)	51 (96.23)	122 (89.70)
46-60	10 (25.64)	01 (2.27)	–	11 (8.09)
Total	**39 (100)**	**44 (100)**	**53 (100)**	**136 (100)**

Source: Field Survey, 1999-2000.

Note: Figures shown in parenthesis refer to the percentage of total Sample women.

Table 5.4. Sex Ratio in the Sample Household

Females / 1000 Males (Group)	*Category of the Sample*			*Total*
	General	*Pregnant*	*Lactating*	
Below 600	07 (17.95)	06 (13.64)	11 (20.75)	24 (17.65)
601-800	07 (17.95)	08 (18.18)	11 (20.75)	26 (19.12)
801-900	–	01 (2.27)	04 (7.55)	05 (3.68)
901-1000	17 (43.59)	13 (29.55)	08 (15.09)	38 (27.94)
Above 1001	08 (20.51)	16 (36.36)	19 (35.86)	42 (31.61)
Total	**39** **(100)**	**44** **(100)**	**53** **(100)**	**136** **(100)**

Source: Field Survey, 1999-2000.

Note: Figures shown in parenthesis refer to the percentage of total Sample women.

The analysis of sex ratio reveals the numerical relationship between women and men, which can be expressed as number of females 1000 males. A ratio of 1000 indicates equal balance of males and females in the population, less than 1000 denotes deficit of women (low sex ratio), and more than 1000 indicates numerical surplus of women (high sex ratio) in the population. Data regarding the sex ratio of the sample households are categorised into five groups below 600 females/1000 males, 601 to 800 females, 801 to 900, 901 to 1000 and above 1001 females per thousands males. Table 5.4 indicates that out of the total 31.61% households have high sex ratio i.e. surplus women while remaining 68.39% households have low sex ratio. It is worth to mention here that all the censuses of India and Uttarakhand since 1872, have recorded relatively smaller number of women, up to 2001 this trend has accentuated in every decades. The numerical imbalance between the sexes and gradual deterioration since the beginning of the 19th century has been the concern of many scholars and as such the sex ratio in any region of India has been a topic of much speculation and investigation. However, the prominent factor for the low sex ratio in this region are:– son preference, unequal treatment given to boys and girls, female infanticide, neglect of female infants, early marriage, death during pregnancy, bad treatment of women and hard work. On contrary this an average, sex ratio in the fully hill districts of Uttarakhand is high because of the out migration of male populating from the villages (Pant, 1996a).

Table 5.5. Educational Level of the Sample

Particular	*Category of the Sample*			*Total*
	General	*Pregnant*	*Lactating*	
Illiterate*	24 (61.54)	24 (54.55)	22 (41.51)	70 (51.47)
Literate*	15 (38.46)	20 (45.45)	31 (58.49)	66 (48.53)
Primary Standard**	06 (40.00)	10 50.00)	14 (45.16)	30 (45.45)
Junior Standard**	05 (33.33)	05 (25.00)	09 (29.03)	19 (28.79)
Intermediate Standard**	03 (20.00)	04 (20.00)	08 (25.81)	15 (22.73)
Graduate and Above**	01 (6.67)	01 (5.00)	–	02 (3.03)
Total	**39** **(100)**	**44** **(100)**	**53** **(100)**	**136** **(100)**

Source: Field Survey, 1999-2000.

* Percentage of the total sample women

** Percentage of the total literature

Note: Figures shown in parenthesis refer to the percentage.

The educational level of the sample women in the villages have been presented in table 5.5. Table indicates that 51.47% sample women were found illiterates. The proportion of illiterate women was varied from 30% in Ghunsera village to

100% Thari and Bharatpur No. 1 villages. The education of 45.45% women was up to primary level. Table 5.5 revels that the women whose education level was junior high school constitute 28.79% in the total literate. It is very considerable feature that the numbers or percentage of literate women has decreased when the level of education increased. The education level of 22.73% women was Intermediate and only 3.03% was Graduate. There were two graduate women in the total samples and they were from village Ramdatt and Chchetrapal. A significant variation was found in the educational level of the sample women in different villages. The study shows that the education level of the sample women in different villages. The study shows that the education level of the sample women was not beyond Junior High School standard in the villages Goshikuan, Chchenigoth, Himmatpur Dotiyal and Haripur Kaliajala. Out of total 136 sample or 66 literates, there were only 15 women (22.73% of the total literates) whose education was Intermediate (Table 5.5).

Agriculture is the basic source of livelihood of the majority of the population in Uttarakhand Himalaya. It is worth to mention that its inhabitants are engaged in more than one occupation because none of occupations provide self-reliant base. In the present study the sample women have been categorised into three main occupations agriculture, service, and labour including routine unavoidable chores of households. Taking all the sample together 98.52% women were engaged in agricultural activities including animal husbandry (Table 5.6). There were only two women in the total sample whose occupation were identified as service and labourer and they were found in village Ramdatt and Thari respectively. It is worth to clear that a sample women of Ramdatt village who was in teaching service was graduate and had no child and a women who was identified as labourer has no personal agricultural land in the village because her husband has given the land in rent basis to immigrants, consequently the family was compelled for labouring.

Table 5.6. Occupational Sructure of the Sample

*Occupations**	*Category of the Sample*			*Total*
	General	*Pregnant*	*Lactating*	
Agriculture and livestock etc.	37 (94.88)	44 (100.00)	53 (100.00)	134 (98.54)
Agriculture and Service	01 (2.56)	–	–	01 (0.73)
Labouring only	01 (2.56)	–	–	01 (0.73)
Total	**39 (100)**	**44 (100)**	**53 (100)**	**136 (100)**

Source: Field Survey, 1999-2000.
* Including household activities.

Note: Figures shown in parentheses refer to the percentage of total Sample.

5.3 Drudgery of the Rural Women

The rural women of Uttarakhand are overburdened with work load. Women participation is found in almost all the rural occupations. Besides all household activities, women role in agricultural operations is very significant and their contribution workout to more than three-fourth of the labour required for agricultural and animal husbandry operations. Consequently the life of rural women in this region is one of the extreme drudgery, misery and deprivation. The women participation in agricultural operations include land preparation, manuring, leveling, sowing, transplanting, weeding, hoeing, applying fertilizers, harvesting, threshing, taking care of crops from animals, winnowing, drying carrying the products from field to home, storage of grains and their by products and so on. The participation of menfolk in agriculture is confined mainly to ploughing of land, irrigation and harvesting. The off farm activities include work relating to rearing of animals, and fetching fodder and fuel wood from forests, rearing of children and old aged, milching cattle, cleaning utensils, stretching new clothes, washing clothes, repairing of old clothes, processing fruits, drying vegetables and grains, grinding and husking of food-grains, cooking, bringing water, knitting, spinning, as well as extending help in marriage, religious and heavy work ceremonies (*Palta*) of neighbourers or relatives. It is observed that in some places particularly remote areas, feeding and grazing animals is done by male members. Average per day working hours of the sample women is categorised into four groups – working below 8 hours, working 12 hours, 16 hours and working about 20 hours and presented in table 5.7. Table 5.7 reveals that only three (2.21%) women of the total 136 samples were working 8 hours a day. It is noticed that among them two women were pregnant in village Khukreta whose works were shared by the family members, and one in village Ramdatt was in teaching service, her husband's cooperation was good as well as they had no child and animals. Overwhelming proportion about 72% of the total sample were spent 16-20 hours a day. This highlights the amount of physical labour that rural women folk have to perform in various activities. This overburdened work, in the absence of proper nutritious diet and health care is bound to create serious health repercussions for the mother and child. The outdoor work are highly time consuming and about 10 hours (62%) out of average daily 16 hours is consumed towards its performance. Remaining time is devoted to indoor activites, which are already mentioned earlier. It noticed that the entertainment hours are very less for the women folk than that of their male counterpart. The working hours of the women for performing the indoor and outdoor activities varies from one season to another. It is observed that the hours of daily work are highest in the rainy season because relatively more crops are grown during this season.

Table 5.7. Working Hours of the Sample

Working Hours Group	*Category of the Sample*			*Total*
	General	*Pregnant*	*Lactating*	
Below 8 Hours	01 (2.56)	02 (4.54)	– –	03 (2.21)
12 Hours	08 (20.51)	10 (22.73)	10 (18.87)	28 (20.59)
16 Hours	24 (61.54)	22 (50.00)	35 (66.04)	81 (59.56)
20 Hours	06 (15.39)	10 (22.73)	08 (15.09)	24 (17.64)
Total	**39 (100)**	**44 (100)**	**53 (100)**	**136 (100)**

Source: Field Survey, 1999-2000.
Note: Figures shown in parenthesis refer to the percentage of total Sample

5.4 Household Income

The economic status of the households certainly depends on the occupational pattern. The annual output (income) of per capita has worked out often summing up the total output from all sources. But for convenience the income sources of the households are classified into three categories such as: 1. Agricultural, livestock etc. 2. Agricultural and service 3. Labouring (Table 5.8). Table reveals that 7.35 households were depend on only agricultural activities while 30.15% households were depend on cultivation, animal rearing, labouring and other activities. Maximum 38.24%, households income sources were agriculture, contractership, and masonry activities. About 20% and 4% households income sources were respectively agriculture, money order, service, and labouring only. Per capita income of each sample has been worked out and grouped into five categories – VLIG (per capita annual income below Rs. 2000), LIG (Rs. 2001 – 3500), MIG (Rs. 3501 – 5000), HIG (Rs. 5001 – 6500) and VHIG (above Rs. 6501) (Table 5.9). Taking all the sample women together,

5.14, 26.47, 28.68, 16.18 and 23.53 percent sample women were respectively in the group of VLI, LI, MI, HI, and VHI. Table reveals that maximum about 60% sample women were below poverty line as their annual income was below Rs. 5000. On the basis of price index for the year 1991–92, the Govt. of India has revised the limit of poverty line as annually Rs. 11000/- per household. During the field study, the question about the sufficiency level was asked from the respondent. The result presented in table 5.10. Table reveals that 50% sample women were self-reliant and rest 50% were dependent on market. Almost similar trend was found in all the sample villages. The one sample village of Bachcham who was complete depend on market and one was self reliant village Bharatpur No. 1.

Table 5.8. Main Income/Output Sources of the Sample

Source	*Category of the Sample*			*Total*
	General	*Pregnant*	*Lactating*	
Agricultural Only	03 (7.69)	03 (6.82)	04 (7.55)	10 (7.35)
Agriculture, Livestock Labouring and Others Only	09 (23.08)	18 (40.91)	14 (26.41)	41 (30.15)
Agriculture, Contract, Masonry etc.	19 (48.72)	14 (31.82)	19 (35.85)	52 (38.24)
Agriculture, Money Order, and Service	06 (15.38)	09 (20.45)	12 (22.64)	27 (19.85)
Labouring Only	02 (5.13)	–	04 (7.55)	06 (4.41)
Total	**39** **(100)**	**44** **(100)**	**53** **(100)**	**136** **(100)**

Source: Field Survey, 1999-2000.

Note: Figures shown in parenthesis refer to the percentage of total Sample Households.

Table 5.9. Economic Level of the Sample

Economic Level	*Category of the Sample*			*Total*
	General	*Pregnant*	*Lactating*	
VLIG (Very Low Income Group)	02 (5.13)	– –	05 (9.43)	07 (5.14)
LIG (Low Income Group)	08 (20.51)	13 (29.55)	15 (28.30)	36 (26.47)
MIG (Moderate Income Group)	09 (23.08)	16 (36.36)	14 (26.42)	29 (28.68)
HIG (High Income Group)	10 (25.64)	05 (11.36)	07 (13.21)	22 (16.18)
VHIG (Very High Income Group)	10 (25.64)	10 (22.73)	12 (22.64)	32 (23.53)
Total	**39** **(100)**	**44** **(100)**	**53** **(100)**	**136** **(100)**

Source: Field Survey, 1999-2000.
Note: Figures shown in parenthesis refer to the percentage of total Sample Households.

Table 5.10. Sufficiency Level of the Sample Households

Levels	*Category of the Sample*			*Total*
	General	*Pregnant*	*Lactating*	
Sufficient	21 (53.85)	20 (45.45)	27 (50.94)	68 (50.00)
Dependent	18 (46.15)	24 (54.55)	26 (49.06)	68 (50.00)
Total	**39** **(100)**	**44** **(100)**	**53** **(100)**	**136** **(100)**

Source: Field Survey, 1999-2000.
Note: Figures shown in parenthesis refer to the percentage of total Sample.

5.5 Height and Weight of the Sample Women

Data on anthropometric measurements of adult Indian women was very scanty. It is during last 15 years that some information has become available through studies done by the National Nutrition Monitoring Bureau (1980). The mean weights and heights of sample women have been grouped and presented in tables 5.11 and 5.12. Table 5.11 reveals that 28% of the total women were below 40 kg weight which can be termed as low weight from pregnancy point of view.

Table 5.11. Body Weight of the Sample

Body Weight Group (in kg)	*Category of the Sample*			*Total*
	General	*Pregnant*	*Lactating*	
Below 35	– –	– –	01 (1.89)	01 (0.73)
36 - 40	11 (28.21)	11 (25.00)	15 (28.30)	37 (37.21)
41 - 45	12 (30.77)	09 (20.45)	16 (30.19)	37 (27.21)
46 - 45	12 (30.77)	17 (38.64)	16· (30.19)	45 (33.09)
Above 51	04 (10.25)	07 (15.91)	05 (9.43)	16 (11.76)
Total	**39 (100)**	**44 (100)**	**53 (100)**	**136 (100)**

Source: Field Survey, 1999-2000.
Note: Figures shown in parenthesis refer to the percentage of total Sample.

About 60% women weight were between 41 to 50 kg while 11.76% women were more than 51 kg weight. Average weight of the sample was 44.29 kg only. Table 5.12 indicates that women's height between 140 to 145 cm were 7.35% which can be termed as short statured. About 55.15% women were between the 151-155 cm heights. This study shows that the weight in reference to height of sample women was very low

Table 5.12. Height of the Sample

Height Group (in kg)	*Category of the Sample*			*Total*
	General	*Pregnant*	*Lactating*	
140 - 145	03 (7.69)	03 (6.82)	04 (7.55)	10 (7.35)
146 - 150	08 (20.51)	14 (31.82)	12 (22.64)	34 (25.00)
151 - 155	21 (53.85)	22 (50.00)	32 (60.38)	75 (55.15)
156 - 160	07 (17.95)	05 (11.36)	05 (9.43)	17 (12.50)
Total	**39 (100)**	**44 (100)**	**53 (100)**	**136 (100)**

Source: Field Survey, 1999-2000.

Note: Figures shown in parenthesis refer to the percentage of total Sample.

which supports the hardworking of the hill women. Average height, weight and Body Mass Index (BMI) of the sample in the villages are presented in table 5.13. Body Mass Index was calculated using the formula weight (kg)/height^2(m). Average BMI varies from 17.79 in village Thari to 20.72 in village Bharatpur No. 1. Similar trend was seen in the general, pregnant and lactating women. Table 5.13 shows the distribution of Body Mass Index.

BMI has been classified in seven groups as defined by James *et al.* (1988). Using BMI < 18.5 as the criteria (optimum) for Chronic Energy Deficiency (CED) 42.54% of the women were found suffer from various degrees of CED (Table 5.14). Among them 1.47% were found to suffer from CED, Grade III (<16.0, severe), 11.76% from CED Grade II (16.01 to 17.0, mild), and 29.41% from CED Grade I (17.01- 18.5, moderate) form of malnutrition. About 56.62% of total women were found to suffer low weight normal and normal. Only one case (0.74%) of the total sample women was found to suffer the obsese Grade I who was belong to Chchetrapal village.

Table 5.13. Average Weight, Height and Body Mass Index (BMI) of the Sample.

Sample Village	Category of the Sample											
	General			*Pregnant*			*Lactating*			*Total*		
	Weight (Kg.)	*Height (cm)*	*BMI (kg/h2m)*	*Weight (Kg)*	*Height (cm)*	*BMI (kg/h2m)*	*Weight (Kg)*	*Height (cm)*	*BMI (kg/h2m)*	*Weight (Kg)*	*Height (cm)*	*BMI (kg/h2m)*
1	2	3	4	5	6	7	8	9	10	11	12	13
1. Goshikuan	41.67	149.00	18.73	39.67	147.67	18.18	38.25	148.25	17.45	39.86	148.31	18.12
2. Khukreta	46.33	154.00	19.50	46.67	152.67	20.86	46.75	153.75	19.51	46.33	153.47	19.96
3. Thari	39.67	117.33	17.50	42.00	149.50	18.81	37.67	148.00	17.06	39.78	138.28	17.79
4. Chchenigoth	41.67	150.67	18.35	39.67	150.67	17.48	41.50	151.75	18.02	40.95	151.03	17.95
5. Bharatput No. 1	48.50	151.50	21.14	51.50	151.00	22.59	41.50	150.00	18.44	47.17	150.83	20.72
6. Himmatpur Dotiyal	44.33	153.00	18.93	38.67	150.00	17.18	44.00	152.50	18.91	42.33	151.18	18.34
7. Ramdatt	46.67	152.33	20.06	47.33	152.33	20.39	44.75	152.75	18.91	46.25	152.47	19.79

Contd.

1	2	3	4	5	6	7	8	9	10	11	12	13
8. Haripur Kaliajala	41.67	153.67	17.64	46.00	153.33	19.54	40.50	152.50	17.40	42.72	153.17	19.29
9. Bhaisori	44.67	152.67	19.59	44.67	15.33	18.97	44.75	152.25	19.30	44.70	152.75	19.29
10. Ghunsera	41.00	150.67	18.05	48.00	153.33	20.41	45.50	153.30	19.18	44.83	152.43	19.21
11. Lakhanarhi	47.00	153.00	20.06	47.67	153.33	19.75	47.00	155.00	19.55	47.22	154.44	19.79
12. Chhetrapal	47.50	156.00	19.52	47.00	150.33	20.93	47.80	150.60	21.08	47.43	153.30	20.51
13. Pachar	49.00	152.67	21.13	46.25	150.75	20.37	46.67	150.67	20.59	47.31	151.36	20.70
14. Bachcham	42.33	149.00	19.12	46.25	152.75	19.79	41.00	143.33	19.10	43.19	148.36	19.34
Total Average	**44.33**	**149.68**	**19.24**	**45.10**	**151.50**	**19.66**	**43.40**	**151.05**	**18.89**	**44.29**	**150.81**	**19.26**

Source: Field Survey, 1999 – 2000.

The mean BMI was 19.26. Seven villages (50%) are below the mean BMI. It is observed that where literacy was low there BMI was also low.

Table 5.14. Average Body Mass Index of the Sample (CED)

Group	*Category of the Sample*			*Total*
	General	*Pregnant*	*Lactating*	
< 16 – CED Grade III (Severe)	–	01 (2.27)	01 (01.89)	02 (1.47)
16.01 – 17.0 CED Grade II (Mild)	06 (15.38)	04 (9.09)	06 (11.32)	16 (11.76)
17.01 – 18.50 CED Grade I (Moderate)	11 (28.21)	11 (25.00)	18 (33.96)	40 (29.41)
18.51 – 20.00 Low Weight Normal	09 (23.08)	09 (20.46)	16 (30.19)	34 (25.00)
20.00 – 25.0 Normal	13 (33.33)	18 (40.91)	12 (22.64)	43 (31.62)
25.01 – 30.0 Obsese Grade I	–	01 (2.27)	–	01 (0.74)
>30.01 Obsese Grade II	–	–	–	–
Total	**39 (100)**	**44 (100)**	**53 (100)**	**136 (100)**

Source: Field Survey, 1999-2000.

Note: Figures shown in parenthesis refer to the percentage of total Sample.

5.6 Fertility Pattern

The mean age at the time of marriage in the Uttarakhand varies from one region to another. It was 15.53 years in the hills (Tripathi, 1980) compared to 18.3 years in the country as a whole in 1981. The percentage of married females in 1981 in in the rural areas for the age group 10-14 years was 7.82% and for the age group 15-19 years was 48.92% (Anon, 1988). Table 5.15 shows that 15.44% women have no children, while 8.82% women have more than 6. About 40% and 35% sample

Table 5.15. Fertility Pattern in the Sample

Particular	*Category of the Sample*			*Total*
Total Birth (in Group) (% of Total)	***General***	***Pregnant***	***Lactating***	
Nil	06 (15.38)	14 (31.82)	–	20 (14.71)
Upto 02	11 (28.21)	11 (25.00)	33 (62.26)	55 (40.44)
Upto 04	18 (46.15)	18 (40.91)	12 (22.64)	48 (35.29)
5 and Above	04 (10.26)	01 (2.27)	08 (15.10)	13 (9.55)
Alive Birth (% of Total)				
Male	60 (53.10)	31 (40.26)	62 (48.44)	153 (48.11)
Female	53 (46.90)	46 (59.74)	66 (51.56)	165 (51.89)
Total Alive	113 (90.4)	77 (91.67)	128 (96.24)	318 (92.98)
Died (% of Total)				
Male	04 (33.33)	03 (42.86)	03 (60.00)	10 (41.67)
Female	08 (66.67)	04 (57.14)	02 (40.00)	14 (58.33)
Total Died	12 (9.60)	07 (8.33)	05 (3.76)	24 (7.02)
Age of Death Time (%)				
< 01 Month	06 (50.00)	02 (28.57)	01 (20.00)	09 (37.50)
2 - 5 Months	05 (41.67)	04 (57.14)	–02 (40.00)	11 (45.84)
6 - 12 Months	–	01 (14.29)	01 (20.00)	02 (8.33)
13 - 16 Months	01 (8.33)	–	01 (20.00)	02 (8.33)

Source: Field Survey, 1999-2000.

Note: Figures shown in parenthesis refer to the percentage of total.

women were having one or two and three or four babies respectively. It is noticed that the average spaceing between the consecutive deliveries was less than 2 years in samples. Data regarding the alive births, died and age of child death time is presented in table 5.15. Table 5.15 reveals that total child bearing women have been given birth to 318 children 165 girl and 153 boys. Total 24 babies were expired during 1998–2000. Among them 83.34% were not survived up to five months. Another table 5.16 shows the incidence of still births, miscarriage and uninduced abortions. In this sample population total 37 cases (27.21%) experienced at least one abortion. About 43.59% of total general, 22.73% of pregnant and 18.87% of total lactating women were suffered from this fetal experience of abortion, still birth. It is primarily due to early marriage of women and partly due to the extremely hard life and harsh condition of work, coupled with nutrition deficiency. Pregnant and lactating women have been widely recognised as a vulnerable section of the society from the health and nutritional point of view. Considerable attention has not been paid to their dietary intake and nutritional status in the region. It is universally accepted that the lactating and pregnant women needed more nutritious food to feed her offspring. The records about the pregnant, lactating and infants care were not incomplete but also poorly maintained. Some oral information about these groups were gathered during the field study. It is noticed that out of total 44 pregnant women about 64% were not vaccinised (Table 5.17). It varied from one village to another, lower vaccination is due to lack of health facilities as well as of awareness. It is noticed that the percentage of women who were vistited a health facility and those who were visited at home by the health workers (ANM) were very low. Data regarding the lactating women is presented table 5.18. Likewise pregnant women 60.38% of lactating women were also not vaccinised during their pregnancy period. Table 5.18 reveals that the 100% deliveries were normal.

Majority of the rural women were unaware of antenatal services even the 90 tablets of iron and folic acid. Out of the total 53 lactating women 88.68% women were delivered the

Table 5.15. Abortion, Still Birth and Miscarriage Incidence Among the Sample

Sl. No.	*Sample Villages*	*Category of the Women*			*Total*
		General	*Pregnant*	*Lactating*	
	1	**2**	**3**	**4**	**5**
1.	Goshikuan	02 (66.67)	–	01 (33.33)	03 (100.00)
2.	Khukreta	02 (50.00	02 (50.00)	–	04 (100.00)
3.	Thari	02 (66.67)	01 (33.33)	–	03 (100.00)
4.	Chchenigoth	02 (66.67)	–	01 (33.33)	03 (100.00)
5.	Bharatpur No. 1	01 (100.00)	–	–	01 (100.00)
6.	Himmatpur Dotiyal	01 (33.33)	01 (33.33)	01 (33.34)	03 (100.00)
7.	Ramdatt	01 (33.33)	01 (33.33)	01 (33.34)	03 (100.00)
8.	Haripur Kaliajala	01 (33.33)	01 (33.33)	01 (33.34)	03 (100.00)
9.	Bhaisorhi	02 (50.00)	–	01 (50.00)	02 (100.00)
10.	Ghunsera	01 (33.33)	01 (33.33)	01 (33.34)	03 (100.00)
11.	Lakhanarhi	01 (50.00)	–	01 (50.00)	04 (100.00)
12.	Cherapal	01 (50.00)	01 (50.00)	–	02 (100.00)
13.	Pachar	–	01 (100.00)	–	01 (100.00)
14.	Bachacham	–	01 (50.00)	01 (50.00)	02 (100.00)
	Grand Total	17 (45.96)	10 (27.02)	10 (27.02)	37 (100.00)
	% of Total Sample	43.59	22.73	18.87	27.21

Source: Field Survey, 1999-2000

Note: Figures shown in parenthesis refer to the percentage of the total cases in the Village.

offspring at home remaining 11.32% were at hospitals. It is noticed during the field study that only complicated delivery cases were admitted to the far flung located hospitals. Table 5.18 shows that 75.45% of the total deliveries were conducted untrained dais and mostly friends and relatives. The percentage of deliveries conducted by untrained persons is more in villages not located in the vicinity of the Primary Health Center or sub-center. It is also noticed that a number of PHCs and sub-centers are running without specialised medical personnels. It is very sad that inspite of large number of trained dais, most deliveries in rural areas of Uttarakhand are still being attended by untrained persons. Such type of care at the time of birth has a major role to play in determining the survival of mother and offspring. Approximately 70% of the total 53 lactating women is the bedding conditions during deliveries were very bad. In most of the families, mothers and their new born baby were not allowed to move out from the fixed separate portion of the room, generally ground floors of the house or even cattlesheds were utilized for this purpose. It is also observed that both the mother and their offspring were not touched by the others i.e. such untouchebility were exist in the villages so far.

Likewise food intake of the 58.49% of lactating women were not healthy, number of restrictions were imposed by the society up to the 11 days. It is enough to know the extent of imposition on the women from one example that milk and vegetables are not allowed during this primary period of 11 days from the birth of baby (*Namkarnasanskar).* Vegetables are considered as cold or *badi* items which are not allowed for a long time of delivery. It is customary in special items porridge-wheat flour mixed with sugar or gur (Jaggary) and bread were given in these days. In the sanitation point of view it is very striking feature that both mother and child would bath after a gap of three days i.e. third, sixth, ninth and eleventh days of the delivery. As a result, mothers and their babies are more vulnerable to suffer various disease and increase the numbers of mortality and morbidity. However,

Table 5.17. Information of Pregnant Women (44 cases)

Villages	*Physical Condition*		*Vaccination*		*Feeling About Health*	
	Good	*Bad*	*Yes*	*No*	*Good*	*Bad*
1	2	3	4	5	6	7
Goshikuan	01 (33.33)	02 (66.67)	01 (33.33)	02 (66.67)	01 (33.33)	02 (66.67)
Khukreta	02 (66.67)	01 (33.33)	02 (66.67)	01 (33.33)	02 (66.67)	01 (33.33)
Thari	01 (25.00)	03 (75.00)	04 (100.00)	–	02 (50.00)	01 (50.00)
Chchenigoth	–	03 (100.00)	01 (33.33)	02 (66.67)	01 (33.33)	02 (66.67)
Bharatpur No 1	01 (50.00)	01 (50.00)	01 (50.00)	01 (50.00)	01 (50.00)	01 (50.00)
Himmatpur Dotiyal	–	03 (100.00)	–	03 (100.00)	–	03 (100.00)
Ramdatt	02 (66.67)	01 (33.33)	02 (66.67)	01 (33.33)	01 (33.33)	02 (66.67)
Haripur Kaliajala	01 (33.33)	02 (66.67)	01 (33.33)	02 (66.67)	01 (33.33)	02 (66.67)

Bhaisorhi	02 (66.67)	01 (33.33)	01 (33.33)	02 (66.67)	01 (33.33)	02 (66.67)
Ghunsera	02 (66.67)	01 (33.33)	01 (33.33)	02 (66.67)	02 (66.67)	01 (33.33)
Lakhanarhi	02 (66.67)	01 (33.33)	02 (66.67)	01 (33.33)	03 (100.00)	–
Chetrapal	02 (66.67)	01 (33.33)	–	03 (100.00)	02 (66.67)	01 (33.33)
Pachar	01 (25.00)	03 (75.00)	–	04 (100.00)	01 (25.00)	03 (75.00)
Bachcham	01 (25.00)	03 (75.00)	–	04 (100.00)	02 (50.00)	02 (50.00)
Grand Total	**18**	**26**	**16**	**28**	**20**	**24**
% Total Villages	**48.91**	**59.09**	**36.36**	**63.64**	**45.45**	**54.55**

Source: Field Survey, 1999-2000.

Note: Figures shown in parenthesis refer to the percentage of total cases in the Village.

Table 5.18. Some Silent Features of the Lactating Women in the Villages (53 cases)

Villages	Vaccination		Delivery Types		Birth Place		Birth Assistant		Bedding During Delivery		Food Pattern During Delivery	
	Yes	No	Normal	Abnormal	Home	Hospital	Non Trained	Trained Doctor	Bad	Good	Healthy	Unhealthy
1	2	3	4	5	6	7	8	9	10	11	12	13
Goshikuan	02 (50.00)	02 (50.00)	04 (100.00)	–	04 (100.00)	–	04 (100.00)	–	03 (75.00)	01 (25.00)	01 (25.00)	03 (75.00)
Khukerta	03 (75.00)	01 (25.00)	04 (100.00)	–	02 (50.00)	02 (50.00)	02 (50.00)	02 (50.00)	03 (75.00)	01 (25.00)	03 (75.00)	01 (25.00)
Thari	03 (100.00)	– –	03 (100.00)	–	03 (100.00)	– –	02 (66.67)	01 (33.33)	02 (66.67)	01 (33.33)	01 (33.33)	02 (66.67)
Chcheni goth	02 (50.00)	02 (50.00)	04 (100.00)	–	04 (100.00)	–	04 (100.00)	–	04 (100.00)	–	01 (25.00)	03 (75.00)
Bharatpur No. 1	02 (100.00)	–	02 (100.00)	–	02 (100.00)	–	02 (100.00)	–	02 (100.00)	–	–	02 (100.00)
Himmat-pur Dotiyal	01 (25.00)	03 (75.00)	04 (100.00)	–	04 (100.00)	–	03 (75.00)	01 (25.00)	02 (50.00)	02 (50.00)	02 (50.00)	02 (50.00)
Ramdatt	01 (25.00)	03 (75.00)	04 (100.00)	–	03 (75.00)	01 (25.00)	03 (75.00)	01 (25.00)	03 (75.00)	01 (25.00)	03 (75.00)	01 (25.00)

Haripur Kaliajala	– –	04 (100.00)	04 (100.00)	–	03 (75.00)	01 (25.00)	03 (75.00)	01 (25.00)	03 (75.00)	01 (25.00)	01 (25.00)	03 (75.00)
Bhaisorhi	01 (25.00)	03 (75.00)	04 (100.00)	–	04 (100.00)	–	02 (50.00)	02 (50.00)	03 (75.00)	01 (25.00)	01 (25.00)	03 (75.00)
Ghunsera	02 (50.00)	02 (50.00)	04 (100.00)	–	02 (50.00)	02 (50.00)	03 (75.00)	01 (25.0)	03 (75.00)	01 (25.0)	02 (50.00)	02 (50.00)
Lakhanarhi	02 (40.00)	03 (60.00)	05 (100.00)	–	05 (100.00)	–	03 (60.00)	02 (40.00)	03 (60.00)	02 (40.00)	02 (40.00)	03 (60.00)
Chetrapal	02 (20.00)	03 (60.00)	05 (100.00)	–	05 (100.00)	–	03 (60.00)	02 (40.00)	02 (40.00)	03 (60.00)	03 (60.00)	02 (40.00)
Pachar	–	03 (100.00)	03 (100.00)	–	03 (100.00)	–	03 (100.00)	–	02 (66.67)	01 (33.33)	01 (33.33)	02 (66.67)
Bachcham	–	03 (100.00)	03 (100.00)	–	03 (100.00)	–	03 (100.00)	–	02 (66.67)	01 (33.33)	01 (33.33)	02 (66.67)
Grand Total	**21**	**32**	**53**	–	**47**	**06**	**40**	**13**	**37**	**16**	**22**	**31**
% of Total Villages	**39.62**	**60.38**	**100.00**	–	**88.68**	**11.32**	**75.47**	**24.53**	**69.81**	**30.19**	**41.51**	**58.49**

Source: Field Survey, 1999-2000.

Note: Figures shown in parenthesis refer to the percentage of total cases in the Village.

such data has not been gathered during the field survey because generally women were concealed to provide these type of information and they did not want to recollect such fetal time.

Contrary to immunization/vaccination pattern among the nursing mothers, about 66% new born babies in the sample villages were immunized regularly and about 34% were not visited the hospitals (Table 5.19). Similarly 58.49% offsprings were breast-feeding and remaining 41.51% were bottle feeded. It is observed that the major causes of bottle-feeding was partially due to the lack of milk producing by mothers and partially mothers were suffered from pregnancy complications. Same table 5.19 also represents the average weight of infants at the time of birth. It is worth to mention that few cases whose weight were taken at the time of birth remaining were depend on the respondent average. Only 24.53% mothers gave birth to infants who weighed more than 2.51 kg while majority (47.17%) of them gave birth to infants who weighed between 2.01 to 2.50 kg and 28.30% infants were below 2 kg weight. The main cause of low birth weight-below 2.50 kg infants constitute 75.47% of the total was poor calorie and protein intake by mothers during the pregnancy in one hand and hard work in difficult terrain on the other.

5.7 Housing and Environmental Sanitation Pattern

The health status of the people in any region largely depends upon the physical quality of the environment. Health is a crucial attribute of human resource and a healthy human population is the most desired national asset. Adequate sanitation and safe potable water are necessary for the prevention of infectious and water born diseases. Inadequacy of the safe drinking water and improper disposal of night soil, solid and liquid wastes leading to polluted environmental conditions and lack of personal and food hygiene have been the major cause of many killer diseases in developing countries including India (Banerji, 1985 and Anon, 1992b). While there

Table 5.19. Information of Offsprings

Villages	*Immunized*		*Offspring*		*Weight of Infants (in kg)*		
	Yes	*No*	*Breast Feeded*	*Bottle Feeded*	*Below 2.0*	*2.01 – 2.50*	*2.51 and above*
1	**2**	**3**	**4**	**5**	**6**	**7**	**8**
Goshikuan	01 (25.00)	03 (75.00)	02 (50.00)	02 (50.00)	02 (50.00)	02 (50.00)	–
Khukreta	04 (100.00)	–	04 (100.00)	–	01 (25.00)	01 (25.00)	02 (50.00)
Thari	03 (100.00)	–	02 (66.67)	01 (33.33)	01 (33.33)	02 (66.67)	–
Chchenigoth	02 (50.00)	02 (50.00)	02 (50.00)	02 (50.00)	02 (50.00)	02 (50.00)	–
Bharatput No. 1	02 (100.00)	–	01 (50.00)	01 (50.00)	–	01 (50.00)	01 (50.00)
Himmatpur Dotiytal	04 (100.00)	–	02 (50.00)	02 (50.00)	01 (50.00)	02 (50.00)	01 (50.00)
Ramdatt	04 (100.00)	–	02 (50.00)	02 (50.00)	–	03 (75.00)	01 (25.00)
Haripur Kaliajala	04 (100.00)	–	02 (50.00)	02 (50.00)	01 (25.00)	02 – (50.00)	01 (25.00)

Contd.

1	2	3	4	5	6	7	8
Bhaisorhi	01 (25.00)	03 (75.00)	03 (75.00)	01 (25.00)	02 (50.00)	01 (25.00)	01 (25.00)
Ghunsera	02 (50.00)	02 (50.00)	02 (50.00)	02 (50.00)	02 (50.00)	01 (25.00)	01 (25.00)
Lakhanarhi	04 (80.00)	01 (20.00)	02 (40.00)	03 (60.00)	02 (40.00)	02 (40.00)	01 (20.00)
Chetrapal	04 (80.00)	01 (20.00)	03 (60.00)	02 (40.00)	–	03 (60.00)	02 (40.00)
Pachar	–	03 (100.00)	02 (66.67)	01 (33.33)	–	02 (66.67)	01 (33.33)
Bachcham	–	03 (100.00)	02 (66.67)	01 (33.33)	01 (33.33)	01 (33.33)	01 (33.33)
Grand Total	**35**	**18**	**31**	**22**	**15**	**25**	**13**
% of Total Villages	**66.04**	**33.96**	**58.49**	**41.51**	**28.30**	**47.17**	**24.53**

Source: Field Survey, 1999-2000.

Note: Figures shown in parenthesis refer to the percentage of total.

exist elaborate arrangement for housing and sanitation in the urban areas, rural housing and sanitation have been of marginal interest of the policy makers. Health surveys conducted in different parts of the country reveal that about 70% of the morbidity and mortality among rural population can be attributed to the direct or indirect effects of poor environmental conditions in the villages (Santhanan, 1989). Realizing the significance of environmental sanitation, particularly of water supply and sanitation, the WHO (1953) expert committee on environmental sanitation recommended provision of adequate supply of water and safe disposal of human excreta (night soil) as essential step for hygienic environmental conditions in rural areas. Even environmental Hygiene Committee of Government of India, as early as in 1984, suggested that measures should be taken to make the provision of safe drinking water supply and sanitation. Moreover, following the recommendations of UN Habitat Conference (1976), UN Water Conference (1977) decided to observe 1981-90 as the "International Drinking Water and Sanitation Decade", which was finally endorsed by 31st UN General Assembly in 1977. According to the resolution passed in the General Assembly, the member states had agreed to provide its population safe drinking water and hygienic waste disposal by the year 1990.

Village-wise data regarding the housing and environmental sanitation is presented in table 5.20. In the sample villages 73.5% households have *pucca* houses while 11.8% of the households were still living in the house made of mud, tatar and thatches (*Kuchcha*) and 14.7% had mixed houses i.e. partially *pucca*. Table reveals that generally *Kuchcha* houses were found in Tarai and Bhabar region. It is due to the non-availability of roof and wall materials in Tarai-Bhabar region and low economic status of the sample households. It is customary that either any economic status of the households he had essentially a *pucca* house in the mountainous region of the study area. Separate cattlesheds were generally found in the sample villages. Courtyards were made by mud, bricks slate and cement. About 63.2% of the total courtyards were in bad condition in terms of level, boundary wall, sanitation etc. while nearly one-third of total (36.81%) were found in good condition. In the rural areas, along with the type of housing, the quality of houses is also greatly affected by the provision of ventilation, sunlight condition, and pest and insects condition etc. The ventilation condition of 47% houses was very bad. The sunlight condition of the majority of the houses (72.2%) was good while about 90% of the total sample houses were suffering from the pests and insects, also effect its inhabitants. Of the total households only 52.2% have used/ sprayed the pesticides and insecticide in their houses to protect themselves and foodgrains from the pests and insects.

In evaluation of the housing condition from the health viewpoint, it is not merely the type or quality of house but its size or room density (persons/room) also plays very important role. As evident from table 5.20, the room density about 8% of the total households was one person/room while the population of 38.3% households was living more than four persons in single room. About 57.4% households have attached kitchen i.e. one corner of any room generally ground floor has utilized for kitchen purpose while 42.6% households have separate kitchens either *pucca* or *kachcha*. It is very serious problem in the villages where about 85.3% and 88.2% households have not bathroom and latrines facilities respectively. Latrines were constructed generally outside the houses. It is observed that only economically well off households had latrine and bathroom facility. As there was no public latrine facility in the villages majority of the households (88.2%) have to go open fields and nearby water streams for latrine. Though, it provides manure, the soil get indiscriminately polluted resulting in heavy infestations with helminthes parasites. Clearing the toilets is problematic due to cultural perception and this discouraged people from having toilets either inside or outside the house.

Lack of safe drinking water and indiscriminate defecation are the major sources of many serious diseases. Table 5.20 dipicts that major source of water supply was public taps, as about 53.7% of the households have mentioned it as the main

Table 5.20. Housing and Sanitation Condition in the Sample Villages

S. No.	Villages	Sample Villages						
		Goshi-kuan	*Khukreta*	*Thari*	*Chche-nigoth*	*Bharat-pur No. 1*	*Himmatpur Dotiyal*	*Ramdatt*
	1	2	3	4	5	6	7	8
1.	**Type of House**							
	Kuchcha	50.00	20.00	60.00	20.00	16.70	–	–
	Pucca	30.00	60.00	10.00	40.00	50.00	90.00	100.00
	Mixed	20.00	20.00	30.00	40.00	33.30	10.00	–
2.	**Courtyard Condition**							
	Good	40.00	30.00	60.00	40.00	16.70	40.00	60.00
	Bad	60.00	70.00	40.00	60.00	83.30	60.00	40.00
3.	**Ventilation**							
	Good	50.00	30.00	30.00	30.00	16.70	50.00	70.00
	Bad	50.00	70.00	70.00	70.00	83.30	50.00	30.00
4.	**Sunlight Condition**							
	Good	90.00	90.00	100.00	80.00	100.00	80.00	70.00
	Bad	10.00	10.00	–	20.00	–	20.00	30.00
5.	**Pets/Insects Condition**							
	Good	–	20.00	–	20.00	–	–	20.00
	Bad	100.00	80.00	100.00	80.00	100.00	100.00	80.00

Contd.

1	2	3	4	5	6	7	8
6. **Use of Pesticides/Insecticides**							
Yes	80.00	100.00	40.00	40.00	16.70	30.00	60.00
No	20.00	–	60.00	60.00	83.30	70.00	40.00
7. **Accommodation Availability (P/room)**							
One	–	–	–	–	–	–	20.00
Two	10.00	30.00	10.00	30.00	16.70	20.00	50.00
Three	50.00	40.00	30.00	20.00	–	40.00	20.00
Four and above	40.00	30.00	60.00	50.00	83.30	40.00	10.00
8. **Type of Kitchen**							
Attached	30.00	20.00	60.00	40.00	83.30	70.00	80.00
Separate	70.00	80.00	40.00	60.00	16.70	30.00	20.00
9. **Bathroom Facility**							
Yes	–	20.00	–	–	16.70	10.00	40.00
No	100.00	80.00	100.00	100.00	83.30	90.00	60.00
10. **Toilet Facility**							
Yes	–	20.00	–	–	16.70	–	40.00
No	100.00	80.00	100.00	100.00	83.30	100.00	60.00
11. **Open Space around the house**							
Good	80.00	100.00	50.00	70.00	100.00	60.00	60.00
Bad	20.00	–	50.00	30.00	–	40.00	40.00

12.	**Source of Drinking Water**							
	Handpump	90.00	100.00	80.00	100.00	–	–	–
	Tap	10.00	–	20.00	–	100.00	100.00	100.00
	Other	–	–	–	–	–	–	–
13.	**Water Disposal Condition**							
	Covered	–	30.00	–	–	–	–	–
	Open	100.00	70.00	100.00	100.00	100.00	100.00	100.00
14.	**Refused Disposal Condition**							
	Pits	10.00	30.00	–	50.00	–	–	20.00
	Open	90.00	70.00	100.0	50.00	100.00	100.00	80.00
15.	**Street Conditions**							
	Good	20.00	30.00	–	40.00	16.67	10.00	60.00
	Bad	80.00	70.00	100.00	60.00	83.30	90.00	40.00
16.	**Proximity of Garbage**							
	Nil	90.00	70.00	100.00	70.00	100.00	90.00	60.00
	Distant	10.00	30.00	–	30.00	–	10.00	40.00
17.	**Garbage Condition**							
	Open	100.00	80.00	100.00	80.00	100.00	100.00	50.00
	Closed	–	20.00	–	20.00	–	–	50.00

Contd.

	Haripur Kaliajala	*Bhaisorhi*	*Ghunsera*	*Lakhanarhi*	*Chchetra-pal*	*Pachar*	*Bachcham*	*Total*
	9	10	11	12	13	14	15	16
1. **Type of House**								
Kuchcha	–	–	–	–	–	–	–	11.8
Pucca	90.00	100.00	80.00	100.00	100.00	100.00	80.00	73.5
Mixed	10.00	–	20.00	–	–	–	–	14.7
2. **Courtyard and Condition**								
Good	20.00	50.00	20.00	40.00	20.00	50.00	20.00	36.8
Bad	80.00	50.00	80.00	60.00	80.00	50.00	80.00	63.2
3. **Ventilation**								
Good	40.00	70.00	50.00	70.00	70.00	70.00	80.00	52.9
Bad	60.00	30.00	50.00	30.00	30.00	30.00	20.00	47.1
4. **Sunlight Condition**								
Good	70.00	60.00	60.00	80.00	70.00	70.00	70.00	77.2
Bad	30.00	40.00	40.22	20.00	30.00	30.00	30.00	22.8
5. **Pets/Insects Condition**								
Good	–	–	–	10.00	20.00	50.00	–	10.3
Bad	100.00	100.00	100.00	90.00	80.00	50.00	100.00	89.7
6. **Use of Pesticides/Insecticides**								
Yes	40.00	60.00	40.00	50.00	60.00	70.00	30.00	52.2
No	60.00	40.00	60.00	50.00	40.00	30.00	70.00	47.8

7. **Accommodation Availability (P/room)**								
One	–	–	20.00	10.00	10.00	50.00	–	**8.0**
Two	–	40.00	30.00	60.00	50.00	40.00	10.00	**28.7**
Three	30.00	30.00	20.00	10.00	30.00	10.00	10.00	**25.0**
Four and above	70.00	30.00	30.00	20.00	10.00	–	80.00	**38.3**
8. **Type of Kitchen**								
Attached	70.00	30.00	100.00	100.00	40.00	40.00	50.00	**57.4**
Separate	30.00	70.00	–	–	60.00	60.00	50.00	**42.6**
9. **Bathroom Facility**								
Yes	–	20.00	–	10.00	30.00	60.00	–	**14.7**
No	100.00	80.00	100.00	90.00	70.00	40.00	100.00	**85.3**
10. **Toilet Facility**								
Yes	20.00	20.00	–	–	20.00	50.00	–	**11.8**
No	80.00	80.00	100.00	100.00	80.00	50.00	100.00	**88.2**
11. **Open Space around the house**								
Good	70.00	80.00	70.00	50.00	50.00	60.00	40.00	**66.2**
Bad	30.00	20.00	30.00	50.00	50.00	40.00	60.00	**33.8**
12. **Source of Drincking Water**								
Handpump	–	–	–	–	–	–	–	**27.2**
Tap	100.00	60.00	–	60.00	100.00	50.00	70.00	**53.7**
Other	–	40.00	100.00	40.00	–	50.00	30.00	**19.1**

Contd.

	9	10	11	12	13	14	15	16
13. **Water Disposal Condition**								
Covered	–	–	100.00	–	20.00	–	–	4.4
Open	100.00	100.0	90.00	100.00	80.00	100.00	100.00	95.6
14. **Resfused Disposal Condition**								
Pits	10.00	20.00	–	20.00	20.00	20.00	10.00	15.4
Open	90.00	80.00	100.00	80.00	80.00	80.00	90.00	84.6
15. **Street Conditions**								
Good	20.00	20.00	30.00	20.00	30.00	20.00	–	22.8
Bad	80.00	80.00	70.00	80.00	70.00	80.00	100.00	77.2
16. **Proximity of garbage**								
Nil	90.00	80.00	70.00	70.00	60.00	50.00	70.00	75.7
Distant	10.00	20.00	30.00	30.00	40.00	50.00	30.00	24.3
17. **Garbage Condition**								
Open	80.00	70.00	70.00	100.00	70.00	10.00	100.00	85.3
Closed	20.00	30.00	30.00	–	30.00	–	–	14.7

Source: Field Survey, 1999-2000.

source of water supply. However, 19.1% of the households were still taking water from open sources such as naula, dhara, streams and canals which is unhygienic and unsafe for drinking purposes. About 27.2% confined to Tarai and Bhabar region households fetched water through hand pumps. It is observed that there were no one treatment plants for water purification in the villages. Open space around the house is influence the health of its members. About 88.2% households have enough open space in the front while remaining 17.8% houses were in very congestion.

The method of waste water disposal in the sample villages was very unhygienic. It is observed that there were no drainage systems in the villages. There were no drains to carry either the rain water or the waste water. The waste water spills around or infront of the houses which promotes the breeding of mosquitoes and files and spread the diseases. About 95.6% of the households disposed of the water in open space while 4.4% have managed to have drains adjacent to their house. These drains carry the waste water to some distance from where it spills over the open space again. Refusal includes several substances in it like ashes, rubbish, stable manure, home, and street sweeping, garbage, night soil of infants, children, sick persons etc. the method of handling of refuse has a strong bearing of sanitary conditions.

A majority of households (84.6%) have dumped the refuse in open space. Remaining 15.4% of the households were put it in the uncovered ditches. It is observed that people were so unaware to sanitation in the villages that not a single households had a proper covered compost pit for dumping the refuse. Streets or path condition of the 77.2% households were not satisfactory. About 75% garbage stores were close to the houses. Among the total garbage stores, about 85.3% were open and only 14.7% were properly covered and located few distance from the house. Hence the condition of environmental sanitation assessed in terms of water and waste disposal have been very unhygienic in the sample villages as a whole without any differences between castes/class and region.

Rural conditions in the Uttarakhand Himalaya are generally marked by compact settlement (*Bakhali*) to the extents that most dwellings have common walls with their neighbours. Such conditions facilitates dissemination of communicable disease. The justa position of houses and cattlesheds, often in single compound or keeping animals in ground floor of the house, is common feature in the sample villages. This unhealthy practices of keeping draught animals in close proximity to human beings is partly taken to be a safeguard from wild animals and shortage of covered space during the winters. It is a result of insanitary conditions produced by the animal urine and dung which may carry pathogens. The visible effect of such practices in causing infection is beyond the scope of this study, albeit their contribution in producing insanitary and unhygienic conditions cannot be connived at. It is noticed that in the Tarai, Bhabar region the quality of construction and building material, the houses are usually built of mud and tatar with grass roof and no stone foundation. Dirty floor and wall brings the member of the family in contact with several disease agents such as parasites and enteropathogenic bacteria. During the rainy seasons, the drafty and leaky dwellers often enhance the prevalence of respiratory infection i.e. common colds. The compact layout further restricts air circulation and sunshine in most dewellings. The hot and humid conditions are ideal for the multiplication of pathogens and several vectors which in turn help in transimitting infectious diseases.

The rural people already suffering from minor aliments may thus become potential hosts to several water born diseases – dysentery, hookworm, hepatitis, typhoid etc. The open drains can be the dangerous source of disease carrying vectors such as houseflies and mosquitoes. During field study of the sample villages it is found that most families in rural areas were generally little conscious of personal hygiene. Use of common towels and drinking cups, carelessness about handkerchief, imperfectly washed dishes and handssoiled with nasal secretion were familiar practices. Diffusion of some infectious diseases could possibly be related to such unhygienic habits.

5.8 Amenities in the Sample Villages

In this chapter few indicators usch as schools, health centers, transport, communication, bank, market, seed and fertilizer store have been included (Table 5.21). About 71.4% have primary school within the village while 14.3% schools are between 1 to 3 km away from the villages. Nearly 14% of the total sample villages have Junior Basic Schools at a distance of more than 5 km. Coeducational High School and Intermediate Colleges are beyond 5 km in 71.4% and 85.7% villages respectively. These distances are formidable barriers in the persuits of girls education. There is no systematic governance of the school and not very unoften, teachers do not attend the schools regularly. Remoteness and fragmented habitations involve exorbitant administrative costs while the schools lack in even the basic facilities like teacher, building, black board, and floor mattings. Nearly 85.7% villages are at a distance more than 5 km from the allopathic hospital and primary health center. A similar distance has to be covered for reaching a maternity center (64.3%). The veterinary service centers are also very far from the villages. The private clinics in the region are so remotely located that the villages can hardly make use of their amenities. In nearly 35.7%, 35.7% and 28.6% villages of the sample study, the clinics are at a distance of 1 to 3, 3-5 and more than 5 kilometers, respectively. Likewise schools, medical institution are also lack in the basic facilities like doctors, medicine, etc. While number of centers are remaining closed. Nearly 35.7% villages are below 1 km distance from the public road while one village (7.2%) Bachcham is situated about 20 km from the road heads. More than 35.7% villages of the sample study have their closest post office and telegraph office at more than 5 kilometers distance. About 64% villages have their nearest bank at more than 5 kilometers. The wholesale market can be reached only after a track of 5 kilometers or more in 64.3% of the total sample villages. Hundred per cent villages have to track more than 5 kilometers distance for seeds and fertilizers. Remaining other facilities are distance of more than 5 kilometers. These accounts of accessibility highlight the constraints of living in the mountainous area of Uttarakhand Himalaya.

Table 5.21. Accessibility of Various Pulic Amenities to the Sample Villages

Item	*With in Village*	*Below 01 km*	*1-3 km*	*3-5 km*	*Above 5 km*
Primary School	10 (71.4)	02 (14.3)	02 (14.3)	–	–
Junior High School	–	01 (7.2)	03 (21.4)	08 (57.1)	02 (14.3)
High School	–	–	02 (14.3)	02 (14.3)	10 (71.4)
Intermediate College	–	–	–	02 (14.3)	12 (85.7)
Allopathic Hospital	–	–	–	02 (14.3)	12 (85.7)
Maternity and Child Welfare Centre	–	–	–	05 (35.7)	09 (64.3)
Primary Health Centre	–	–	–	02 (14.3)	12 (85.7)
Private Clinic	–	–	05 (35.7)	05 (35.7)	04 (28.6)
Veterinary Hospital	–	–	–	02 (14.3)	12 (85.7)
Public Road	–	05 (35.7)	08 (57.1)	–	01 (7.2)
Post Office	–	–	04 (28.6)	05 (35.7)	05 (35.7)
Telegraph Office	–	–	–	09 (64.3)	05 (35.7)
Bank	–	–	–	05 (35.7)	09 (64.3)
Whole Sale Market	–	–	–	05 (35.7)	09 (64.3)
Seed/Fertility Store	–	–	–	–	14 (100.00)

Source: Field Survey, 1999-2000

Note: Figures shown in parenthesis refer to the percentage of total.

5.9 Hygiene Pattern

Likewise environmental sanitation, sense of hygiene or awareness towards the hygiene also play an important role to determine the health status of the people. Awareness generally depends upon the educational status and economic level and training in particularly. To measure the hygiene pattern among the sample few indicators (daily bath, daily brush, washing hands before meal, soap use and cleaning frequency of nails) have been included which were gathered during the door to door survey. Categorywise data regarding the personal hygiene is presented in table 5.22. Out of the total sample surveyed 41.18% brush their teeth daily. It varies 10% in village Haripur Kaliajala to 80% in Chchenigoth village. It is also worth to mention that brush mean cleaning of teeth by any means. Villagers use wood (Neam, Timru etc.), coal and specific grass for brushing their teeth. Few of them were used ready-made powder or paste. It is very considerable that out of the total 136 samples only 30.88% women took bath daily. It also similarly varies from 10% to 80% in the same villages. About 80.88% women were washed their hands before taking meal while 19.12% were took food by dirty hands which is totally unhygienic. Majority (98.53%) of the sample women were using soap for washing the cloths, bed cover, bed sheets etc. Nearly 93% women were cut their nails monthly while 5.88 and 0.74% were cleans their nails by bimonthly and weekly respectively (Fig. 5.2).

5.10 Food Habits

As it is well-known fact that food is the main source of nourishment for human body, the food is therefore, defined as a substance, which yields heat to energy for building up of new tissues and for repairing wornout tissue as well as for the regulation of the body process. Without proper nutritious food one cannot get the desired physical, mental, social and emotional status. The main source of nourishment for a human body is food, it is called nutrients, available in the foods in different amounts. Health, nutritious food and a balance diet are inter dependent. Nutrition has to be translated into food to meet the needs of the body. The requirement of nutrition is however different according to the age, sex, and occupation. In the present study region the daily energy requirement for general women with moderate work is 2225 kcal, pregnant women with moderate work is 2525 kcal and nursing or lactating women with moderate work is 2700 kcal have been taken as standard requirement (Tables 5.30-5.32). Food items taken by the women have been converted into various nutrient – protein, fat, carbohydrates, mineral and vitamins.

Table 5.22. Personal Hygiene Pattern of the Sample

Particular		*Category of the Sample*			*Total*
	Responses	*General*	*Pregnant*	*Lactating*	
Daily Bath	Yes	17 (43.59)	18 (40.91)	21 (39.62)	**56 (41.18)**
	No	22 (56.41)	26 (59.09)	32 (60.38)	**80 (58.82)**
Daily Brush	Yes	12 (30.77)	13 (29.55)	17 (32.08)	**42 (30.88)**
	No	27 (69.23)	31 (70.45)	36 (67.92)	**94 (69.12)**
Washing Hands before Meal	Yes	33 (84.62)	37 (84.09)	40 (75.47)	**110 (88.88)**
	No	06 (15.38)	07 (15.91)	13 (24.53)	**26 (19.12)**
Soap Use	Yes	39 (100.00)	43 (97.73)	52 (98.11)	**134 (98.53)**
	No	–	01 (2.27)	01 (1.89)	**02 (1.47)**
Nails Cleaning Frequency	Monthly	35 (89.74)	41 (93.18)	51 (96.23)	**127 (93.38)**
	Half Monthly	03 (7.69)	03 (6.82)	02 (3.77)	**08 (5.88)**
	Weekly	01 (2.56)	–	–	**01 (0.74)**

Source: Field Survey, 1999-2000.

Note: Figures are shown in parenthesis refer to the percentage of total sample.

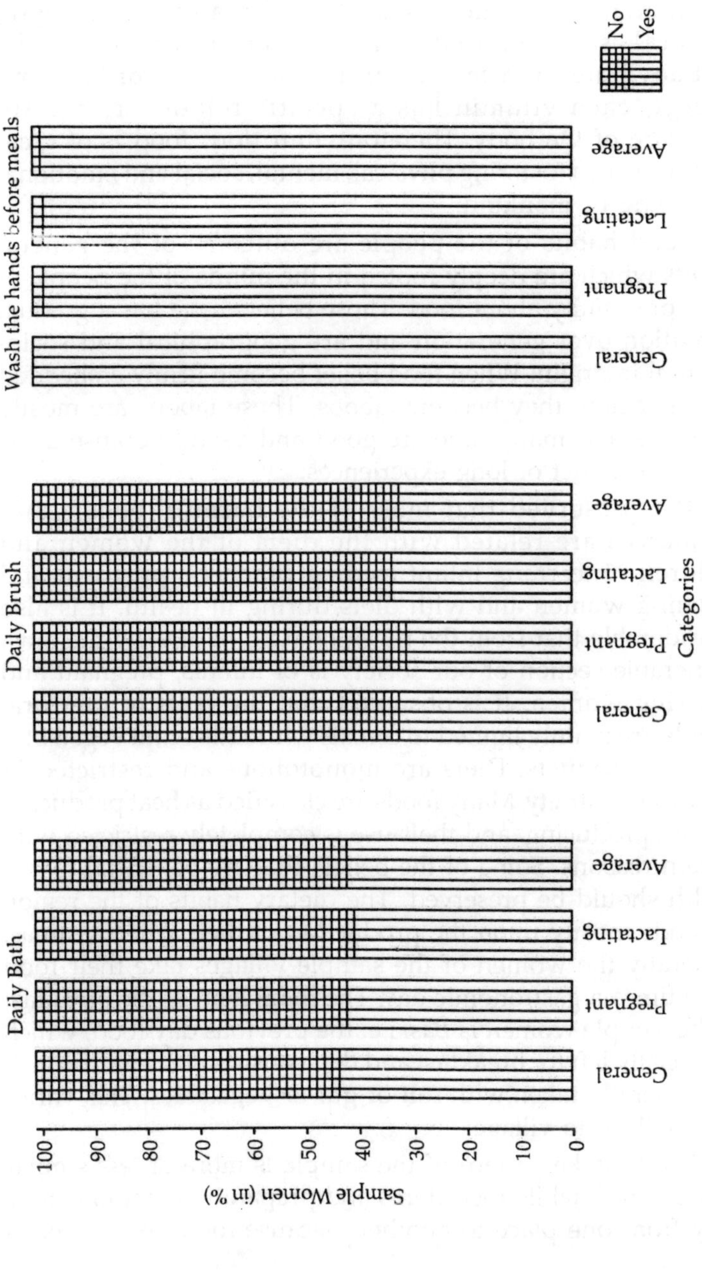

Fig. 5.2. Personal Hygiene Pattern in the Sample Women.

These nutrients have a specific part of its own to play in the human body such as protein is mainly for growth, mineral salts regulates the function of the body, carbohydrates and fats aid in the production of heat and energy, each vitamin has a specific relation to certain structure of the body. Therefore, nutritious food is of great importance in fostering physical, mental, social and emotional wellbeing of mankind.

Food habits of the people are outcome of the general beliefs which are deeply rooted in the minds of the people of any community about food. Those beliefs have has a gradual evolution over generation and are geographical and socio-cultural in origin. When food belief become firmly embedded in the society they become taboos. These taboos are mostly harmless and many time are good and useful because these are the product of long experiences.

It is observed that most of the harmful beliefs and prejudices are related with the diets of the women and children concerning infant feeding practices, pregnant and lactating women and with diets during ill health. It is also considerable that from the nutritional point of view the most vulnerable section of our society is of infants, pregnant and lactating women. It is observed that the diets of the rural people are mainly limited to cereals with little or no vegetables or milk products. Diets are monotonous and restricted in nature and variety. Many foods are classified as heat producing or cold producing, and their use is completely restricted with certain reasons. Some of the beliefs that are beneficial to our health should be preserved. The dietary habits of the region depends mostly upon the production of the particular areas. Generally the women of the sample villages take their food three times a gastronomic day. The main item of the breakfast of the sample women is *Basi* i.e. the previous day food, which is specially left for breakfast and that consists of chapatti which are generally taken with salt or gur or vegetables. This varies from village to village.

Food intake pattern of the sample is more or less similar to the region while food items and preparation methods may vary from one place to another. Because food item depends on the availability of raw food while preparation methods depends on the tradition. The main items for lunch (*Bhat*) are boiled rice and pulse or vegetables. It varies from season to season and also depend upon the availability of the kind of cereals, pulses and vegetables. Chapatti are not taken with lunch. At super, items are chapatti and vegetable with the products of milk and curd are taken as additional food items. Chapaties or rotis are generally made of wheat and madua (ragi) flour separately, wheat and madua flour mixed (*lesuwa/ lesu*), grinded pulses especially urd/gahat put inside the wheat flour (*beruwa*). Among from pulses, gram, soyabean, lentil, pegion-pea, bhat (black soyabean), gahat, urd, malka etc. are generally consumed but poor families or for a change people took kari (*jholi*), grinded gahat (*dubke*), rice mixed with pulses (*khichari*), rice mixed with curd (jaula), or mixed with grinded gahat (rajaru), bhatti bari, muguri, churkani etc. Vegetables (tapkiya) in the day time are occasionally or seasonally consumed. In the evening children take stake meal otherwise they take salt mixed bread either with tea, chatni, gur, ghee or vegetable. It is not taken by matured persons. People take dinner in the form of bread with vegetables. Flesh products are occasionally consumed. Fried meals as puri, kachchauri, haluwa, bare, khee etc are taken on the occasions of festivals and other ceremonies. The milk product consumption also depends on availability and are mostly seasonal (rainy). Fruits consumption depends upon its availability also and are mostly regional and seasonal.

During the course of field study it was noticed that 39% women were regularly taking fast (*upwas*) a particular day, which determine the health status of rural women also heavy work load coupled with fast (*upwas*) affect their health status adversely. Categorywise fast pattern is depicted in table 5.23. It is noticed that only women of Thari and Bachchem villages were not taking fast. Generally two fast in a year on the occasions of Mahashivratri and Krishna Janmasthami were taken by all adult people in the region. As evident from table 5.24 that out of the total samples 19.85% were smokers (bidi & tobacco) and 2.94% were both smoker and drinkers (country made liquor). It is notice that drinking the liquor is traditionally recognise among the tribal women while maximum lower caste women were habitual in smoking the bidi and tobacco. Taking intoxicants and smoking bidi & tobacco not only affects the mother's health but also injurious for their offspring. Majority of the sample are non-vegetarian. Categorywise dietary pattern in the sample villages is presented in table 5.25 and figure 5.3.

Table 5.23. Fast (*Upwas*) Pattern Among the Sample

Responses about Taking fast	*Category of the Sample*			*Total*
	General	*Pregnant*	*Lactating*	
Yes	15 (38.46)	19 (43.18)	20 (37.74)	**54** **(39.71)**
No	24 (61.54)	25 (56.82)	33 (62.26)	**82** **(60.29)**
Total	**39** **(100.00)**	**44** **(100.00)**	**53** **(100.00)**	**136** **(100.00)**

Source: Field Survey, 1999-2000.
Note: Figure shown in parenthesis refer to the percentage of total Sample.

Table. 5.24. Smoking/Intoxication Pattern Among the Sample

Habits	*Category of the Sample*			*Total*
	General	*Pregnant*	*Lactating*	
Smoking	07 (17.95)	10 (22.73)	10 (18.87)	**27** **(19.85)**
Non Smoking	29 (74.36)	34 (77.27)	42 (79.26)	**105** **(77.21)**
Smoking & Drinking	03 (7.69)	–	01 (1.87)	**04** **(2.94)**
Total	**39** **(100.00)**	**44** **(100.00)**	**53** **(100.00)**	**136** **(100.00)**

Source: Field Survey, 1999-2000.
Note: Figure shown in parenthesis refer to the percentage of total Sample.

Out of the total sample 46.32% women had their food twice and 53.68% thrice in a gastronomic day (Fig. 5.3). Though, breakfast includes in almost full meal as they were often engaged in strenuous works. As evident from table 5.25-49.26, 27.94 and 15.44% women had milk, curd and ghee daily while 22.06, 21.33 and 22.06% women did not consumed respectively these items even occasionally (Fig. 5.3). It is observed during the fields study that there were no differences between the pregnant, nursing and general women for the edible items intake point of view. It is well-known fact that milk is most balanced and important diet for health particularly for pregnant and lactating women. Since the study indicates that an overwhelming proportion of the sample women was deprived of these items. Thus, one can imagine the poor health condition of the women in the study region.

Likewise daily pulses intake accounts for only 5.15% of the total sample women while 17.64, 34.56, 36.77 and 5.88% respectively were taking pulses four times per week, two times/week, weekly and monthly (Table 5.25 and Fig. 5.3). Pulses are another important source of nutrients particularly for protein. Out of total 136 sample women 32.35% and 61.65% were vegetation and non-vegetarian respectively. Out of total non-vegetarian 16.30, 48.91 and 34.79% women were consumed flesh products respectively weekly, bi-monthly and occasionally. It is very considerable that 96.32% women have consumed green vegetable monthly. Only 2.21 and 1.47% were taking green vegetable weekly and daily respectively (Fig. 5.3). Green vegetables are also important source of vitamins, the deficiency of which causes various nutrition deficiency diseases. It is also worth to mention that in the rainy and winter seasons people consumed green vegetable twice even thrice in a day but not regularly. Some of the green vegetables like palak (spinach) were prohibited for lactating women in some villages of the region. A study done by the author shows that only 37.09% households had milk, curd and ghee throughout the year (Pant, 1998).

Table 5.25. Food Pattern Among the Sample

Items/Particular Frequency		*Category of the Sample*			*Total*
		General (39 No.)	*Pregnant (44 No.)*	*Lactating (53 No.)*	
1		2	3	4	5
Meal Day	: Two time	21 (53.85)	21 (47.73)	21 (39.62)	63 (46.32)
	Three time	18 (46.15)	23 (52.27)	32 (60.38)	73 (53.68)
Milk	: Daily	15 (38.46)	22 (50.00)	30 (56.60)	67 (49.26)
	Occassionally	13 (33.33)	13 (29.55)	12 (24.53)	39 (28.68)
	Nil	11 (28.21)	09 (20.45)	10 (18.87)	30 (22.06)
Curd	: Daily	10 (25.64)	13 (29.55)	15 (28.30)	38 (27.94)
	Occassionally	18 (46.15)	21 (47.73)	30 (56.60)	69 (50.74)
	Nil	11 (28.21)	10 (22.72)	08 (15.10)	29 (21.32)
Ghee	: Daily	04 (10.26)	07 (15.91)	10 (18.87)	21 (15.44)
	Occassionally	25 (64.10)	27 (61.36)	33 (62.26)	85 (62.50)
	Nil	10 (25.64)	10 (22.73)	10 (18.87)	30 (22.06)
Pulse	: Daily	01 (2.56)	02 (4.55)	04 (7.55)	07 (5.15)
	4 times/week	09 (23.08)	06 (13.64)	09 (16.98)	24 (17.65)
	2 times/week	12 (30.77)	15 (34.09)	20 (37.73)	47 (34.56)
	Weekly	14 (35.90)	20 (45.45)	16 (30.19)	50 (36.76)
	Monthly	03 (7.69)	01 (2.27)	04 (7.55)	08 (5.88)
Habit	: Vegetarian	13 (33.33)	16 (36.36)	15 (28.30)	44 (32.35)
	Non-Vegetarian	26 (66.67)	28 (63.64)	38 (71.70)	92 (67.65)

Contd.

1		2	3	4	5
Flesh (% of non-vegetarian):					
	Weekly	04 (15.38)	05 (17.86)	06 (15.79)	**15** **(16.30)**
	Half Month	09 (34.62)	14 (50.00)	22 (57.89)	**45** **(49.92)**
	Occasionally	13 (50.00)	09 (32.14)	10 (26.32)	**32** **(34.78)**
Green Veget-able	: Monthly	37 (94.89)	42 (95.45)	52 (98.11)	**131** **(96.32)**
	Weekly	–	2 (4.55)	01 (1.89)	**03** **(2.21)**
	2 times/week	02 (5.15)	–	–	**02** **(01.47)**

Source: Field Survey, 1999-2000.

Note: Figures shown in parenthesis refer to the percentage of total Sample.

5.11 Food Intake Pattern

The diet survey of the selected sample women in the sample villages of the study region is carried out through oral questionnaire and weighment methods. In oral questionnaire survey of the raw food consumed the previous day was noted and an weighment method survey the food intake to be prepared for mid day and night were measured in the morning and the evening, respectively. Food items were measured in local units *nali, ser, paw* and then converted into grams and milligrams. Afterwards, the data collected through both were added and that were analysed and therefore the possibility of errors was minimum.

The diet of the study region is primarily based on cereals. Taking together all the 136 sample, approximately the per capita, per day cereal intake was 389.29 grams which is 11.53% less than the standard requirement of 440 grams (Fig. 5.29). In fifty per cent villages the cereal intake was found less than the regional average while per head/day cereal intake of general women was 399.7 grams, pregnant women 391.26 and lactating women was 388.08 grams (Tables 5.26, 5.27 and 5.28).

Categorywise cereal intake is presented in tables 5.26 to 5.29. Per capita daily intake of pulses was only 23.18 grams which is 48.49% less than the standard requirement of 45 grams. It varies from 15.1 grams in village Ghunsera to 46.9 grams in Khukreta. The per capita daily consumption of pulses was found only 23.96 grams in general category women while 23.75 and 21.88 grams were found in pregnant and lactating women category, respectively. The per capita daily vegetable consumption in the region was 41.21 grams which is 78.31% lower than the standard requirement of 190 grams (including root, leafy and other vegetables). The Categorywise vegetable intake was 44.24 grams by general, 40 grams by pregnant and 39.39 grams by the lactating category. Similar trend was found in all the villages and categories. In the study region, the consumption of ghee and cooking oil per capita per day was found 17.58 grams which is 56.05% less than the 40 grams standard requirement. It is because of their poverty and low purchasing capacity. In general category the per capita per day ghee and cooking oil intake was 18.46 grams, while 17.54 and 16.74 grams were consumed by the women of pregnant and lactating categories, respectively.

The average intake of milk products per capita per day was found 81.01 grams, which is 46% lower than the 150 grams standard requirement. Lowest 61.31 grams milk was consumed by the general category women while 83.18 and 87.82 grams intake were found among the pregnant and lactating categories women. The consumption of fruits in the study region is seasonal and occasional. Apart from the fruits produced in the village itself, they are also supplied from urban areas. The average fruits consumption per capita daily is 174.14 grams. About 175.71, 188.93 and 170.7 grams per capita daily fruits consumption were found in general, pregnant, and lactating categories respectively. The physical environment of the region is very suitable for tropical and temperate fruit cultivation. In the study region average intake of the sweet items gur, mishree, sugar etc. per capita per day was 33.29 grams which is 10.97% more than the 30 grams standard

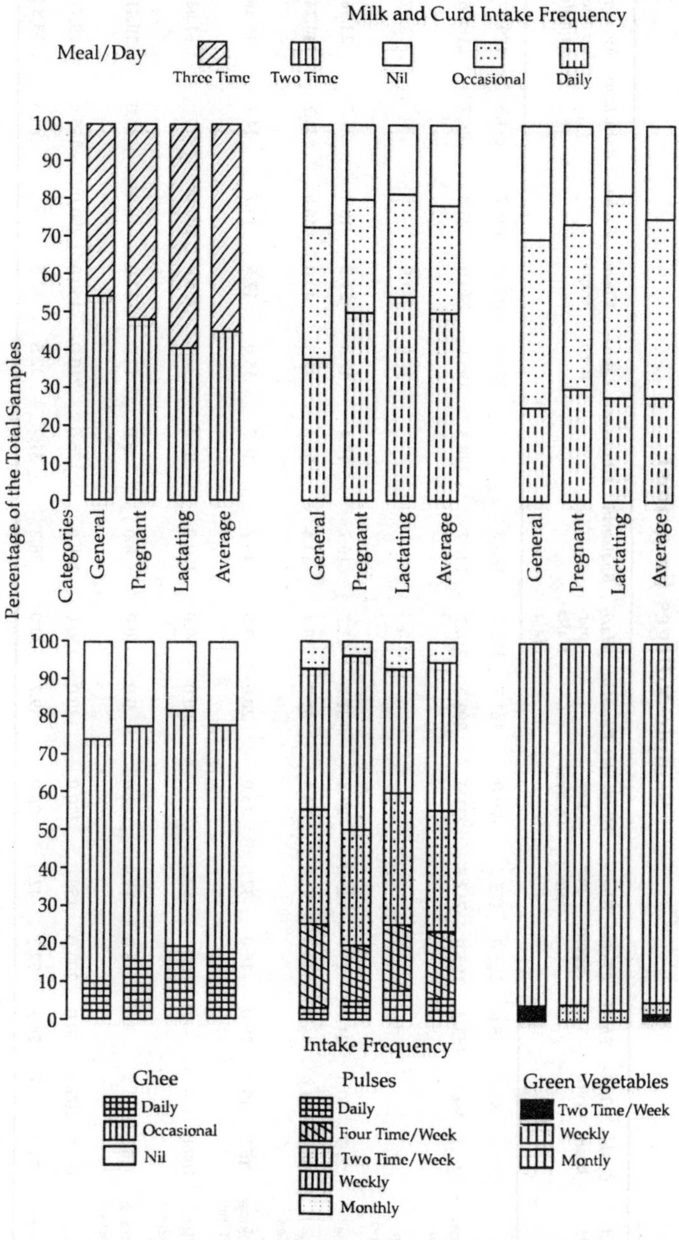

Fig. 5.3. Food Intake Pattern in the Samples Women.

Table 5.26. Average Per Head Per Day Food Consumption of General Category Women in the Sample Villages (in grams)

Food stuff	*Goshi-kuan*	*Khuk-reta*	*Thari*	*Chche-nigoth*	*Bharat-pur No. 1*	*Himmat-pur Dotiyal*	*Ramdatt*	*Hari-pur Kalia-jala*	*Bhaisorhi*	*Ghunsera*	*Lakha-narhi*	*Chche-trapal*	*Pachar*	*Bachcham*	*Average of the sample*
Rice	211.7	83.3	175.0	205.0	175.0	170.0	161.7	181.7	166.7	190.0	207.5	200.0	191.7	193.3	179.47
Wheat flour	166.7	366.7	183.3	195.0	212.5	231.0	203.3	214.7	191.7	188.3	195.0	230.0	228.3	226.7	216.66
Ragi/ Mandua	–	–	–	–	–	–	–	–	–	–	37.5	12.5	–	–	3.57
Pulses	21.7	50.0	21.7	25.0	25.0	23.4	31.7	21.7	16.7	13.4	17.5	27.5	18.4	21.7	23.96
Vege-tables	58.3	51.6	46.7	48.4	32.5	28.3	61.7	35.4	43.4	53.4	41.5	40.0	40.0	38.2	44.24
Cooking oil/Ghee	15.7	40.0	15.0	16.0	32.5	15.0	20.0	13.3	16.7	10.7	15.0	17.5	16.7	14.3	18.46
Milk Products	100.0	–	–	–	50.0	–	200.0	50.0	100.0	83.3	–	175.0	100.0	–	61.63
Spices & Others	10.00	15.8	9.0	8.0	11.0	12.0	9.0	10.0	8.0	9.0	12.0	12.0	9.0	11.0	10.41
Fruits	155.0	205.0	80.0	200.0	150.0	220.0	180.0	150.0	160.0	175.0	210.0	150.0	250.0	175.0	175.71
Sweets	31.7	51.7	26.7	27.3	42.5	26.0	39.7	30.0	28.3	31.7	32.5	42.5	35.0	28.3	33.85

Source: Field Survey, 1999-2000.

Table 5.27. Average Per Head Per Day Food Consumption of Pregnant Category Women in the Sample Villages (in grams)

Food stuff	*Goshi-kuan*	*Khuk-reta*	*Thari*	*Chche-nigoth*	*Bharat-pur No. 1*	*Himmat-pur Dotiyal*	*Ramdatt*	*Hari-pur Kalia-jala*	*Bhaisorhi*	*Ghunsera*	*Lakha-narhi*	*Chche-trapal*	*Pachar*	*Bachcham*	*Average of the sample*
Rice	196.7	150.0	221.2	193.3	160.0	133.3	178.3	186.7	185.0	203.3	200.0	183.3	166.5	198.7	182.59
Wheat flour	191.7	191.7	202.5	185.0	242.5	198.3	228.3	230.0	200.0	240.0	168.3	213.0	186.5	220.0	207.01
Ragi/ Mandua	–	–	–	–	–	–	–	–	–	–	33.3	–	–	–	2.38
Pulses	46.7	43.3	29.9	25.1	27.5	15.0	26.6	20.0	15.1	18.3	21.7	15.0	12.5	15.9	23.75
Vege-tables	46.7	45.0	43.7	38.3	41.0	27.7	41.6	41.1	41.6	53.4	37.4	26.7	36.7	39.2	40.0
Cooking oil/Ghee	21.7	35.0	15.0	18.3	35.0	12.3	16.7	12.3	11.7	13.3	16.7	9.3	14.7	13.5	17.54
Milk Products	–	133.3	–	133.3	112.5	75.0	133.3	125.0	100.0	116.7	66.7	–	50.0	118.7	83.18
Spices & Others	13.5	12.5	11.0	9.5	13.0	8.0	11.0	11.0	11.0	8.0	11.0	9.0	8.0	9.0	10.39
Fruits	175.0	150.0	60.0	150.0	160.0	175.0	210.0	210.0	180.0	210.0	250.0	175.0	210.0	150.0	188.93
Sweets	28.3	50.0	36.2	21.7	42.0	25.0	36.7	30.0	28.3	35.0	36.0	28.3	35.0	31.7	33.17

Source: Field Survey, 1999-2000.

Table 5.28. Average Per Head Per Day Food Consumption of Lactating Category Women in the Sample Villages (in grams)

Food stuff	*Goshi-kuan*	*Khuk-reta*	*Thari*	*Chche-nigoth*	*Bharat-pur No. 1*	*Himmat-pur Dotiyal*	*Ramdatt*	*Hari-pur Kalia-jala*	*Bhaisorhi*	*Ghunsera*	*Lakha-narhi*	*Chche-trapal*	*Pachar*	*Bachcham*	*Average of the sample*
Rice	160.0	156.2	233.3	198.7	–	126.2	192.5	166.2	163.7	167.5	173.0	198.0	170.0	188.3	163.83
Wheat	217.5	256.2	141.7	198.7	327.5	232.5	228.7	221.2	211.7	237.5	190.0	239.0	196.0	203.3	221.54
Ragi/ Mandua	–	–	–	–	–	–	–	–	–	–	40.0	–	–	–	2.86
Pulses	33.6	47.5	25.0	25.3	20.0	17.2	19.2	23.9	14.9	13.7	14.0	18.6	16.7	16.7	21.88
Vege-tables	51.2	55.0	33.3	39.9	27.5	29.0	38.7	33.6	41.2	46.2	38.0	41.0	43.4	33.4	39.39
Cooking oil/Ghee	20.0	36.2	11.7	17.5	15.0	9.2	12.5	13.7	16.2	12.5	19.0	16.6	18.7	15.7	16.74
Milk Products	75.0	137.5	–	100.0	137.5	150.0	118.7	112.5	62.5	102.5	95.0	80.0	58.3	–	87.82
Spices & Others	12.5	13.5	13.0	11.5	10.0	11.0	10.0	9.0	12.0	8.0	9.0	8.0	10.0	8.0	10.39
Fruits	190.0	175.0	90.0	175.0	175.0	200.0	165.0	175.0	220.0	150.0	150.0	200.0	175.0	150.0	170.7
Sweets	37.0	45.0	23.3	36.2	46.5	23.2	337.0	26.2	30.0	30.0	32.0	31.0	36.0	30.0	32.91

Source: Field Survey, 1999-2000.

Table 5.29. Average Per Head Per Day Food Consumption of All Categories Women in the Sample Villages (in grams)

Food stuff	*Goshi-kuan*	*Khuk-reta*	*Thari*	*Chche-nigoth*	*Bharat-pur No. 1*	*Himmat-pur Dotiyal*	*Ramdatt*	*Hari-pur Kalia-jala*	*Bhaisorhi*	*Ghunsera*	*Lakha-narhi*	*Chche-trapal*	*Pachar*	*Bachcham*	*Average of the sample*
Rice	189.5	129.8	209.9	199.0	55.8	143.2	177.5	178.2	171.8	186.8	193.5	193.8	176.1	193.4	**171.31**
Wheat	192.0	271.5	175.5	192.7	260.8	220.6	220.1	222.0	201.1	221.9	184.4	227.4	203.6	216.7	**215.04**
Ragi/ Mandua	–	–	–	–	–	–	–	–	–	–	36.9	4.2	–	–	**2.94**
Pulses	33.9	46.9	25.5	25.1	24.2	18.5	25.9	21.8	15.5	15.1	17.7	20.4	15.9	18.1	**23.18**
Vege-tables	52.1	50.5	41.2	42.2	33.7	28.4	47.3	36.7	42.1	51.0	38.9	35.9	40.0	36.9	**41.21**
Cooking oil/Ghee	19.1	37.0	13.9	17.3	27.5	12.2	16.4	13.1	14.8	12.2	16.9	14.5	16.7	14.5	**17.58**
Milk Products	58.3	90.0	–	77.8	100.0	125.0	150.7	95.8	87.5	100.8	53.9	85.0	69.4	39.6	**81.01**
Spices & Others	12.0	13.9	11.0	9.7	11.3	10.3	10.0	10.0	10.3	8.3	10.7	9.7	9.0	9.3	**10.39**
Fruits	173.3	176.7	76.7	175.0	161.7	198.0	185.0	178.3	186.6	178.3	203.3	175.0	211.7	158.63	**174.14**
Sweets	32.3	48.9	28.7	28.4	43.67	24.7	36.9	28.7	28.8	32.2	33.5	33.9	35.6	30.0	**33.29**

Source: Field Survey, 1999-2000.

etc. were generally consumed in tea and porridges. The average consumption of condiments and spices per capita per day was 10.39 grams. It was noted during the study that the consumption of condiments and spices were similar among all the categories in the sample villages. It is clear from the table 5.25 that per head daily intake of vegetables ghee, cooking oil, meat products, fruits is very inadequate. It is also observed that its inhabitants particularly women were not aware about the essential intake of other food items such as pulses, vegetables, fruits etc. Because of this ignorance they consumed more cereals that other items. In the food intake point of view, there is no much more difference between the general, pregnant and lactating categories women in the region. It is also observed that among the sample women that they were totally ignorant about the additional and nutritious food requirements during the pregnancy and nursing periods even menstrual periods.

5.12 Nutrients Intake Pattern

Food items taken by the women have been converted into various nutrients – protein, fat, carbohydrates, energy, calcium, phosphorous, iron, carotene (vitamin A), thiamine (vitamin B_1), riboflavin (Vitamin B_2), niacin, (nicotinic acid) and ascorbic acid (vitamin C) with the help of Food Composition Tables and then compared with the standard requirement for each category general, pregnant and lactating women determined by the ICMR experts (Gopalan *et al.*, 1993). Categorywise nutrients intake per capita per day of 136 women in the 14 villages has been analysed. Taking together all the sample approximately except iron, thiamine and niacin, the consumption of all other important nutrients was below the standard requirement (Table 5.33). The pattern of nutrients intake is presented in tables 5.30 to 5.33 and figures 5.4 to 5.7. Out of total energy intake 70-80% is drawn from cereals. Remaining energy intake depends on other foods-pulses, vegetables, fruits and milk and which are consumed seasonally and very nominal.

In all the sample, the average energy intake per capita per day was found 1942.2 kcal which is 21.78% below the standard requirement (2483 kcal*). It varies 1734.7 kcal in village Himmatpur Dotiyal to 2320.02 kcal in village Khukreta. The average energy intake in all the villages of the study region was found below the standard requirement. The per head per day energy intake of general category women was found 1957.99 kcal which is 12% below the standard requirement of 2225 kcal. Similarly per capita daily energy intake of pregnant and lactating women was – 23.09% and 29.02% below the standard requirement of 2525 kcal and 2700 kcal, respectively. Categorywise energy intake in the sample villages is presented in tables 5.30-33 (Figure 5.5). Almost three quarters (71%) of the villages, the consumption of energy intake was found less than 2000 kcal.

The average per capita, per day protein intake was found 49.25 gm which is 20.56% below the standard requirement of 62 grams. It varies the 43.54 grams in village Thari to 58.01 grams in village Khukreta which are below the standard requirement. The protein intake by general women was found 49.42 grams, 48.77 grams by the pregnant women and 49.71 grams by the lactating women which are 1.16%, 24.97% and 30.96% respectively below the standard requirement of 50, 65 and 72 grams. In all the villages the average consumption of protein was found below the standard (Table 5.33). The per capita daily protein intake the general category women in Khukreta, Ramdatt, Chhetrapal and Pachar villages was more than the standard requirement because of high consumption of wheat flour in the diet. Remaining fell short by 4.78% in general women of village Haripur Kaliajala to 43.11% in lactating women of village Thari (Tables 5.30-5.33).

The average fat intake per capita per day was found 29.81 grams which is 6.84% below the standard requirement of 32 grams. It varies from 20.55 grams in Thari village to 52.09

* It is (2483 kcal) average of the standard requirement of general (2225) pregnant (2525) and lactating (2700 kcal) categories.

grams which is 6.84% below the standard requirement of 32 grams. It varies from 20.55 grams in Thari village to 52.09 grams in village Khukreta (Table 5.33). The per head per day fat intake by general women was found 29.96 grams while 30.11 and 29.62 grams by pregnant and lactating women respectively which are 48.85% and 0.38% more and 30.96% less than the standard requirement of 20, 30 and 45 grams respectively. On an average only in 21% villages the consumption was found above the standard requirement. These villages are Khukreta, Bharatpur No. 1 and Ramdatt. It is the result of more production and more consumption of milk and oil seeds.

In the study region, average carbohydrates intake was found 363.37 grams per head per day which is 15.5% below the standard requirement (430 grams). It varies from 329.83 grams in village Himmatpur Dotiyal to 398.82 grams in Khukreta village. On an average all the villages were found below the standard requirement (Table 5.33). The per head daily consumption of carbohydrates by general women was found 370.01 grams by pregnant women was 363.84 and 285.37 grams by lactating women which are 13.95, 15.39 and 16.66 per cent below the standard requirement.

Carbohydrate intake by each category in the villages is presented in tables 5.3 to 5.32. Out of the total 14 sample villages, six (43%) villages, the intake was noticed below the regional average. Table 4.30 shows that the carbohydrates intake was found 0.35% above the standard requirement in general category of Khukreta village. The average per capita daily calcium intake was found 544.52 mg in the region which is 31.94% below the standard requirement of 800 gm. It varies from 332.51 mg in village Thari to 761.61 mg in Ramdatt village. Table 5.30 shows that only 4 villages (28%) are below the regional average. However all villages fall short by 4.8% to 58.41% from the normal requirement. Due to different standard requirements for different category the average per head per day calcium intake of general category was found 40.61% above from the standard requirement of 400 mg while

41.57% and 39.36% below calcium intake was noticed in pregnant and lactating women respectively from the standard requirement of 1000 mg. Tables 5.30-5.32 show the per head daily intake of calcium by each category in the sample villages (Figures 5.4 to 5.7).

In the sample villages the average iron intake per capita per day was found 33.59 mg which is 1.79% above the standard requirement of 33 mg. It varies 26.23 mg in village Thari to 47.46 mg in village Khukreta (Table 5.33). The per head daily intake of 50% villages was found above the standard requirement. These villages are Goshikuan, Khukreta, Himmatpur Dotiyal, Ramdatt and Haripur Kaliajala, Ghunsera and Chchetrapal. The average per head per day iron intake of general and lactating category women was found respectively 20% and 12.37% above the standard requirement of 30 mg while the daily iron intake in pregnant category women was found 13.95% below from the standard requirement of 38 mg. Category wise iron intake in the villages is presented in Tables 5.30-5.32.

In the sample villages of the region, the average phosphorus intake per capita per day was found 1299.38 mg which is 7.19% below the standard requirement of 1400 mg. It varies 1095.92 mg in village Thari to 1534.98 mg in village Khukreta. Only two (14.28%) out of fourteen villages, per head daily phosphorus intake was above the standard. These villages are Khukreta and Ramdatt. The main source of phosphorus is cereals and cereals are the main food of the villagers. As however, majority of the villages fall short from the standard requirement. Similarly, the per head daily intake of phosphorus in all the general, pregnant and lactating women categories was 8.64%, 7.33% and 5.59% below the standard requirement of 1400 mg. Tables 5.30-5.32 show the per head per day intake of phosphorus by each category in the sample villages.

In the study region the carotene (vitamin A) intake is unsatisfactory because the consumption of per capita per day was 795.37 μg in average which is 72.23% below the standard requirement of 2867 μg. It varies 563.44 μg in village Thari to 1381.95 μg in village Khukreta. The per head intake of carotene in all the sample villages was found short by 51.80% to 80.35% Similarly the intake of carotene in the all categories was also found below the standard. The per head per day carotene intake is presented in tables 5.30 to 5.33 and figures 5.4 to 5.7.

In the study region, thiamine intake in average was 1.68 mg per head per day which is 34.4% above the standard requirement of 1.25 mg. In all the category of the sample villages of the region of daily consumption of thiamine (vitamin B_1) was found above the standard requirement (Table 5.33).

The average riboflavin (vitamin B_2) intake was 0.68 mg per capita daily which is 53.10% below the standard requirement of 1.45 mg. It also varies 0.62 mg in village Thari to 1.0 mg in village Bharatpur No. 1. In all the villages of the region the consumption was found below the standard requirement. The per head per day intake of riboflavin in general category was 0.79 mg, in pregnant 0.68 mg and 0.72 mg intake was found in lactating category women which is respectively 39.23, 54.67 and 53.55% below the standard requirements of 1.3, 1.5 and 1.55 mg. The per head per day intake of riboflavin in the villages is presented in tables 5.30 to 5.33 and figures 5.4 to 5.7.

In the sample villages, the average niacin (nicotinic acid) intake was found 17.62 mg which is 11.52% above the standard requirement of 15.8 mg. It varies from 16.41 mg in village Himmatpur Dotiyal to 18.91 mg in Khukreta village. On an average all the sample villages of the region, the consumption of niacin was found above the standard requirement. Although the per head per day intake by lactating women was fund only 0.91% below the standard (Table 5.32).

Green vegetables and fruits are the main source of vitamin C (ascorbic acid). In the study region its average intake was found 53.03 mg which is 11.62% fall short from the standard requirement of 60 mg. The per head/day intake of vitamin C, only three villages were found above the standard requirement. It varies from 32.76 mg in village Thari to 71.25

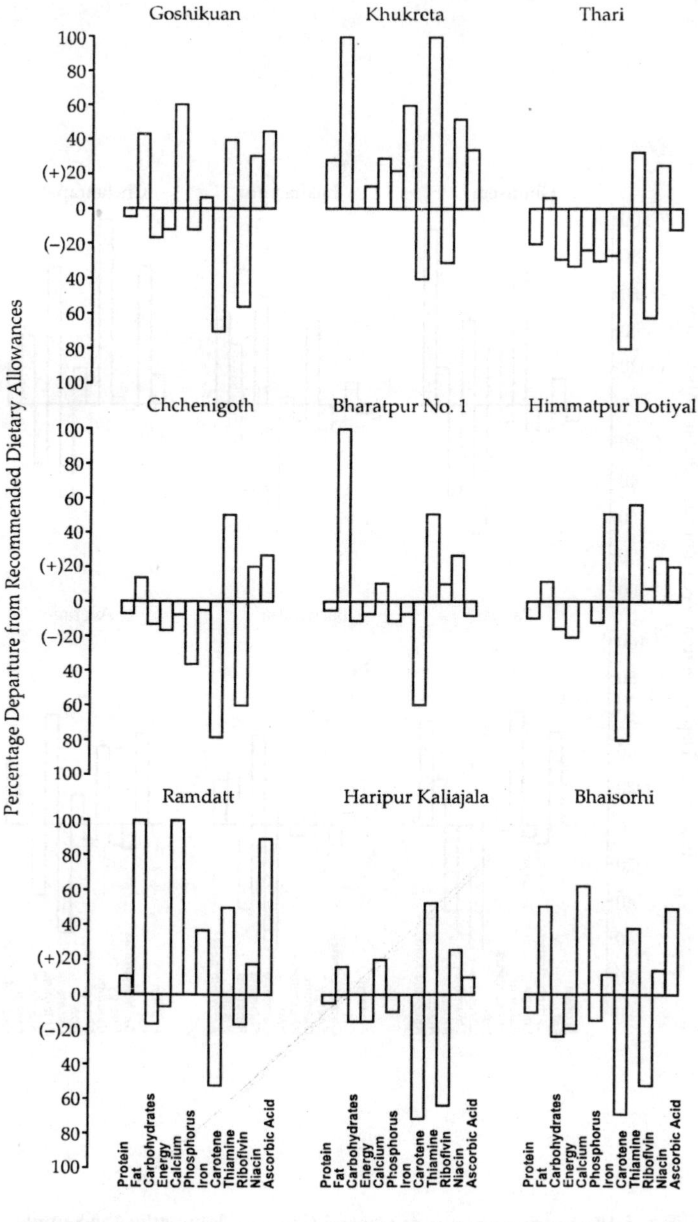

Fig. 5.4A. Nutrition Status of General Category Women in the Sample Villages.

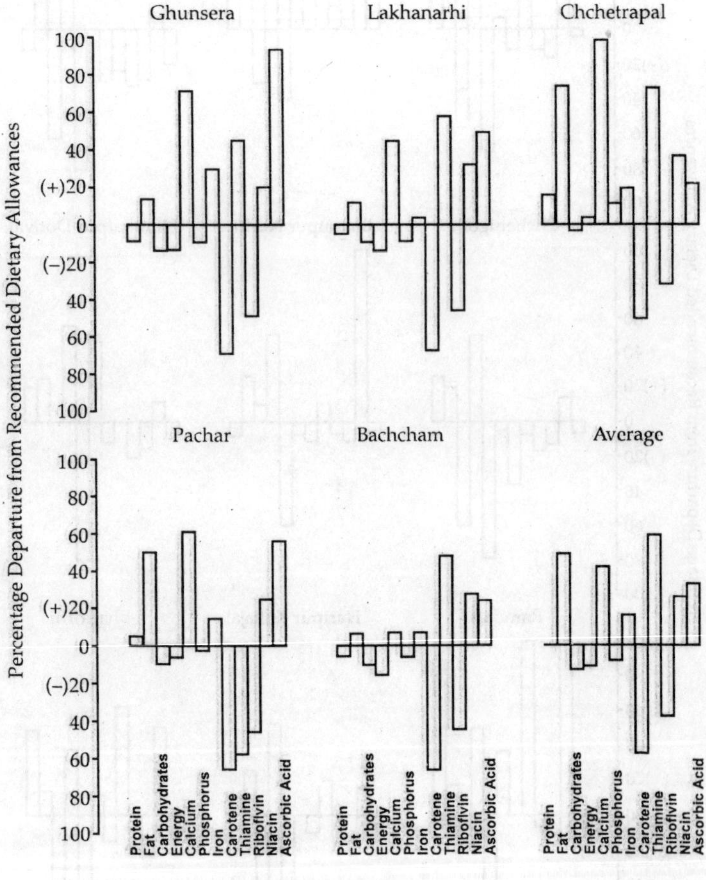

Fig. 5.4B. Nutrition Status of General Category Women in the Sample Villages.

Table 5.30. Per Head Per Day Nutrient Intake Pattern of General Category Women in the Sample Villages.

Nutrients	Recommended Dietary Allowance (RDA)	Goshikuan		Khukreta		Thari		Chchenigoth		Bharatpur No. 1	
		Actual Intake	Percentage Departure from RDA (+) (–)	Actual Intake	Percentage Departure from RDA (+) (–)	Actual Intake	Percentage Departure from RDA (+) (–)	Actual Intake	Percentage Departure from RDA (+) (–)	Actual Intake	Percentage Departure from RDA (+) (–)
1	2	3	4	5	6	7	8	9	10	11	12
Protien	50.0 gm	46.69	-6.62	65.01	+30.02	41.07	-17.86	45.33	-9.34	47.51	-4.98
Fat	20.0 gm	28.57	+42.85	51.19	+155.95	21.35	+6.75	22.41	+12.05	42.76	+113.80
Carbohydrates	430.0 gm	357.06	-16.96	431.50	+0.35	321.36	-25.26	366.83	-14.69	366.54	-14.76
Energy	2225.0 kcal	1893.81	-14.88	2444.91	+9.88	1641.69	-29.22	1850.13	-16.85	2051.55	-7.80
Calcium	400.0 mg	624.40	+56.10	514.72	+28.68	323.07	-19.23	367.25	-8.19	442.78	+10.70
Phosphorus	1400.0 mg	1206.14	-13.85	1712.03	+22.29	1056.89	-24.51	880.37	-37.12	1240.83	-11.37
Iron	30.0 mg	32.00	+6.67	47.04	+56.80	23.16	-22.80	28.07	-6.43	28.06	-6.47
Carotene	2400.0 μg	767.23	-68.03	1374.63	-42.72	565.10	-76.45	586.32	-75.57	1118.70	-53.39
Thiamine	1.10 mg	1.52	+38.18	2.22	+101.82	1.45	+31.82	1.62	+47.27	1.63	+48.18
Riboflavin	1.30 mg	0.61	-53.08	0.86	-33.85	0.52	-60.00	0.56	-56.92	1.43	+10.00
Niacin	14.0 mg	17.91	+27.93	21.40	+52.86	17.49	+24.93	17.26	+23.28	17.33	+23.78
Ascorbic acid	40.0 mg	58.59	+46.48	53.17	+32.93	35.39	-11.53	50.18	+25.45	36.16	-9.60

Contd.

Nutrients	Recommended Dietary Allowance (RDA)	Himmatpur Dotiyal		Ramdatt		Haripur Kaliajala		Bhaisorhi		Ghunsera	
		Actual Intake	Percentage Departure from RDA (+) (–)	Actual Intake	Percentage Departure from RDA (+) (–)	Actual Intake	Percentage Departure from RDA (+) (–)	Actual Intake	Percentage Departure from RDA (+) (–)	Actual Intake	Percentage Departure from RDA (+) (–)
1	2	13	14	15	16	17	18	19	20	21	22
Protien	50.0 gm	47.20	-5.60	55.63	+11.26	47.61	-4.78	45.24	-9.52	45.70	-8.60
Fat	20.0 gm	22.47	+12.35	40.66	+103.30	23.56	+17.80	29.38	+46.90	22.55	+12.75
Carbohydrates	430.0 gm	360.99	-16.05	361.89	-15.84	358.84	-16.55	329.07	-23.47	348.13	-19.04
Energy	2225.0 kcal	1834.90	-17.53	2078.19	-6.60	1848.45	-16.92	1782.98	-19.87	1796.39	-19.26
Calcium	400.0 mg	399.82	-0.05	935.66	+133.92	472.34	+18.09	632.10	+58.03	672.34	+68.09
Phosphorus	1400.0 mg	1246.58	-10.96	1444.82	+3.20	1250.13	-10.71	1199.21	-14.34	1206.01	-13.86
Iron	30.0 mg	45.23	+50.77	41.29	+37.63	29.97	-00.10	32.95	+9.83	37.85	+26.17
Carotene	2400.0 μg	614.09	-74.41	1080.99	-54.96	630.89	-73.71	776.74	-67.64	620.80	-74.13
Thiamine	1.10 mg	1.68	+52.73	1.68	+52.73	1.65	+50.00	1.52	+38.18	1.53	+39.09
Riboflavin	1.30 mg	1.38	+6:15	1.08	-16.92	0.62	-67.69	0.62	-52.31	0.62	-52.31
Niacin	14.0 mg	18.00	+28.57	16.96	+21.14	17.54	+25.29	15.96	+14.00	16.68	+19.14
Ascorbic acid	40.0 mg	48.23	+20.58	76.61	+91.53	43.45	+8.63	60.68	+51.70	75.15	+87.88

Contd.

Nutrients	Recommended Dietary Allowance (RDA)	Lakhanarhi		Chchetrapal		Pachar		Bachcham		Average of the Sample	
		Actual Intake	Percentage Departure from RDA (+) (–)	Actual Intake	Percentage Departure from RDA (+) (–)	Actual Intake	Percentage Departure from RDA (+) (–)	Actual Intake	Percentage Departure from RDA (+) (–)	Actual Intake	Percentage Departure from RDA (+) (–)
1	2	23	24	25	26	27	28	29	30	31	32
Protien	50.0 gm	47.16	-5.68	59.01	+18.02	51.59	+3.18	47.46	-5.68	49.42	-1.16
Fat	20.0 gm	22.50	+12.50	36.55	+82.75	30.26	+51.30	21.49	+7.45	29.69	+48.45
Carbohydrates	430.0 gm	395.83	-7.95	415.83	-3.30	390.66	-9.15	375.67	-12.63	370.01	-13.95
Energy	2225.0 kcal	1975.55	-11.21	2265.61	+1.83	2063.67	-7.30	1885.04	-15.28	1957.99	-12.00
Calcium	400.0 mg	567.07	+41.77	833.41	+108.35	653.92	+63.48	435.02	+8.76	562.42	+40.61
Phosphorus	1400.0 mg	1267.98	-9.43	1559.73	+11.41	1384.22	-1.13	1251.93	-10.58	1279.06	-8.64
Iron	30.0 mg	30.63	+2.10	35.77	+19.23	35.31	+17.70	33.56	+11.87	34.35	+14.5
Carotene	2400.0 μg	621.75	-74.09	977.64	-59.27	794.89	-66.88	591.57	-75.35	794.38	-66.90
Thiamine	1.10 mg	1.74	+58.18	1.91	+73.64	1.77	-60.91	1.71	+55.45	1.69	+53.64
Riboflavin	1.30 mg	0.64	-50.77	0.84	-35.38	0.72	-44.62	0.62	-52.30	0.79	-39.23
Niacin	14.0 mg	18.25	+30.36	19.38	+38.43	18.82	+34.43	18.49	+32.07	17.96	+28.29
Ascorbic acid	40.0 mg	59.66	+49.15	49.48	+23.70	64.58	+61.45	51.51	+28.78	.54.49	+36.23

Source: Field Survey, 1999-2000.

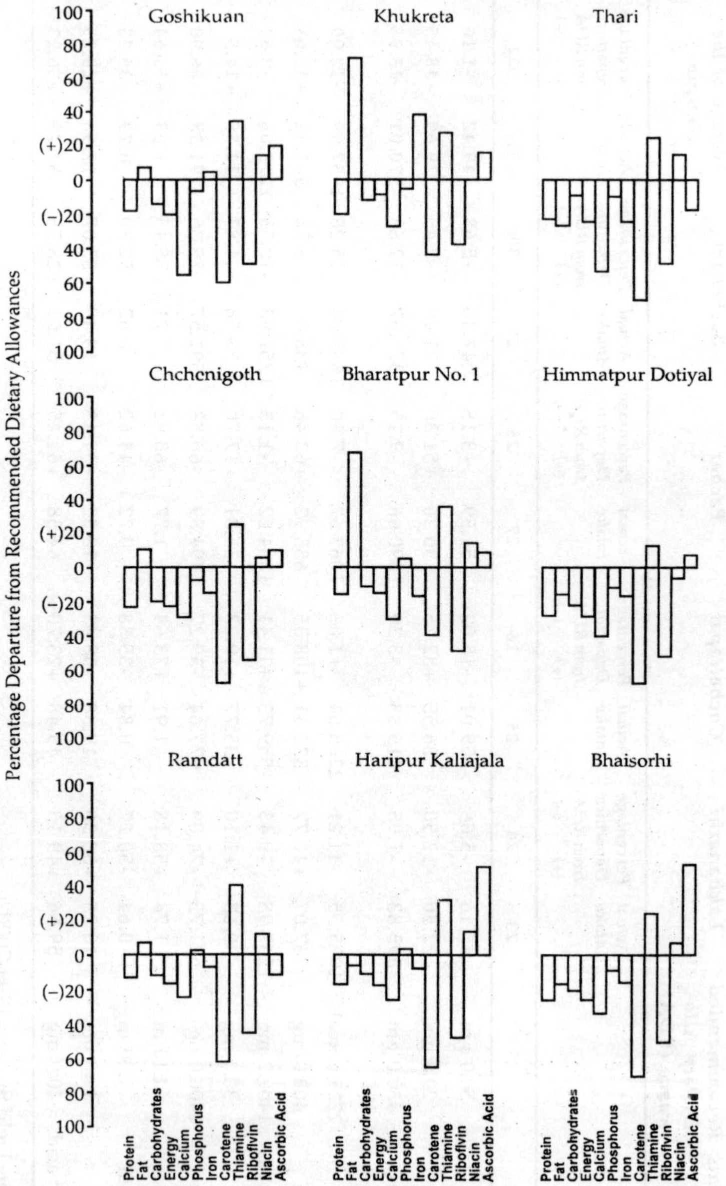

Fig. 5.5A. Nutrition Status of Pregnant Category Women in the Sample Villages.

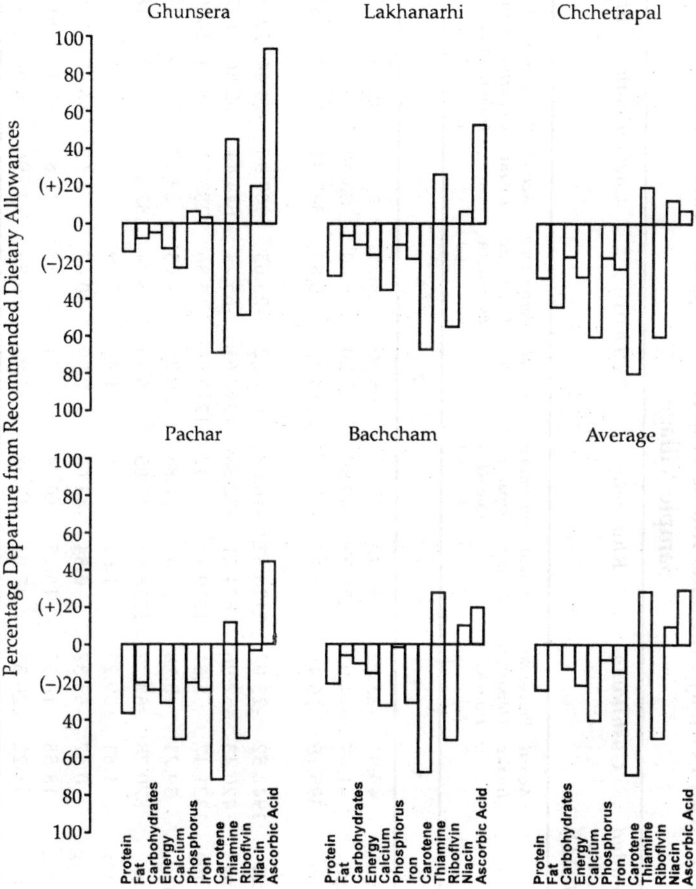

Fig. 5.5B. Nutrition Status of Pregnant Category Women in the Sample Villages.

Table 5.31. Per Head Per Day Nutrients Intake Pattern of Pregnant Category Women in the Sample Villages

Nutrients	*Recommended Dietary Allowance (RDA)*	*Goshikuan*		*Khukreta*		*Thari*		*Chchenigoth*		*Bharatpur No.1*	
		Actual Intake	*Percentage Departure from RDA (+) (–)*	*Actual Intake*	*Percentage Departure from RDA (+) (–)*	*Actual Intake*	*Percentage Departure from RDA (+) (–)*	*Actual Intake*	*Percentage Departure from RDA (+) (–)*	*Actual Intake*	*Percentage Departure from RDA (+) (–)*
1	2	3	4	5	6	7	8	9	10	11	12
Protien	65.0 gm	49.91	-23.22	47.37	-27.12	48.59	-25.25	49.17	-24.35	53.90	-17.08
Fat	30.0 gm	31.47	+4.9	50.99	+69.97	22.20	-26.00	33.48	+11.60	50.29	+67.63
Carbohydrates	430.0 gm	395.15	-16.48	356.47	-17.10	383.33	-10.85	345.33	-19.69	381.086	-11.19
Energy	2525.0 cal	1942.52	-23.07	2120.32	-16.03	1927.72	-23.65	1907.96	-24.44	2218.95	-12.12
Calcium	1000.0 mg	420.43	-57.96	674.21	-32.58	347.61	-65.24	644.44	-35.56	627.91	-37.21
Phosphorus	1400.00 mg	1321.47	-5.61	1310.13	-6.42	1219.98	-12.86	1283.31	-8.34	1429.96	+2.14
Iron	38.0 mg	39.21	+3.18	52.40	+37.84	29.25	-23.03	29.42	-22.58	31.34	-17.53
Carotene	2400.0 µg	870.78	-63.72	1318.85	-47.05	606.20	-74.74	878.30	-63.40	1318.51	-45.06
Thiamine	1.30 mg	1.81	+39.23	1.61	+23.85	1.66	+27.69	1.57	+20.77	1.81	+39.23
Riboflavin	1.50 mg	0.67	-55.33	0.84	-44.00	0.59	-60.67	0.65	-56.67	0.74	-50.67
Niacin	16.00 mg	18.58	+16.13	16.15	+0.94	18.74	+17.13	16.85	+5.13	+18.27	+4.19
Ascorbic acid	40.0 mg	48.22	+20.55	47.03	+17.58	31.91	-20.23	45.96	+14.90	43.21	+8.03

Contd.

Nutrients	*Recommended Dietary Allowance (RDA)*	*Himmatpur Dotiyal*		*Ramdatt*		*Haripur Kaliajala*		*Bhaisorhi*		*Ghunsera*	
		Actual Intake	*Percentage Departure from RDA (+) (–)*	*Actual Intake*	*Percentage Departure from RDA (+) (–)*	*Actual Intake*	*Percentage Departure from RDA (+) (–)*	*Actual Intake*	*Percentage Departure from RDA (+) (–)*	*Actual Intake*	*Percentage Departure from RDA (+) (–)*
1	2	13	14	15	16	17	18	19	20	21	22
Protien	65.0 gm	41.58	-36.03	54.00	-16.92	53.46	-21.59	47.26	-27.29	55.01	-15.37
Fat	30.0 gm	23.19	-22.7	32.97	+9.90	28.11	-6.30	25.05	-16.50	28.25	-5.83
Carbohydrates	430.0 gm	301.96	-29.78	385.98	-10.24	381.48	11.28	350.90	-18.40	406.01	-5.57
Energy	2525.0 cal	1598.83	-36.68	2084.95	-17.43	2018.32	-20.74	1839.65	-27.14	2123.22	-15.91
Calcium	1000.0 mg	490.60	-50.94	690.25	-30.96	726.61	-27.34	645.00	-35.50	752.61	-24.74
Phosphorus	1400.00 mg	1124.14	-19.70	1432.99	+2.36	1426.01	+1.86	12.62.94	-9.79	1467.50	+4.79
Iron	38.0 mg	27.04	-28.89	34.02	-10.47	33.99	-10.55	31.42	-17.32	39.11	+2.92
Carotene	2400.0 µg	611.66	-74.51	876.94	-63.46	747.87	-68.84	674.39	-71.90	746.44	-68.90
Thiamine	1.30 mg	1.43	+10.00	1.76	+35.38	1.76	+35.38	1.56	+20.00	1.88	+44.62
Riboflavin	1.50 mg	0.61	-59.33	0.75	-50.00	0.75	-50.00	0.66	-56.00	0.77	-48.67
Niacin	16.00 mg	14.49	-14.94	18.89	+15.56	18.64	+16.50	17.06	+6.63	19.72	+23.25
Ascorbic acid	40.0 mg	44.01	+10.03	53.71	-15.73	63.70	+59.25	59.72	+49.30	75.40	+88.50

Contd.

Nutrients	Recommended Dietary Allowance (RDA)	Lakhanarhi		Chchetrapal		Pachar		Bachcham		Average of the Sample	
		Actual Intake	Percentage Departure from RDA (+) (–)	Actual Intake	Percentage Departure from RDA (+) (–)	Actual Intake	Percentage Departure from RDA (+) (–)	Actual Intake	Percentage Departure from RDA (+) (–)	Actual Intake	Percentage Departure from RDA (+) (–)
1	2	23	24	25	26	27	28	29	30	31	32
Protien	65.0 gm	46.54	-28.40	43.69	-32.78	41.18	-36.65	51.10	-21.38	48.74	-25.02
Fat	30.0 gm	27.96	-6.80	15.73	-47.57	23.87	-20.43	28.03	-6.57	30.11	+0.38
Carbohydrates	430.0 gm	380.94	-11.41	351.63	-18.23	331.53	-22.90	377.13	-12.30	363.84	-15.39
Energy	2525.0 cal	1975.58	-21.76	1723.31	-31.75	1716.15	-32.03	1990.76	-21.16	1942.02	-23.09
Calcium	1000.0 mg	669.61	-33.04	353.53	-64.65	493.91	-50.61	642.87	-35.71	584.26	-41.57
Phosphorus	1400.00 mg	1249.91	-10.72	1154.43	-17.54	1103.61	-21.17	1376.73	-1.66	1297.37	-7.33
Iron	38.0 mg	26.18	-31.11	29.96	-21.16	29.03	-23.61	25.39	-33.18	32.70	-13.95
Carotene	2400.0 μg	749.03	-68.79	432.93	-81.96	632.14	-73.66	710.82	-70.38	798.20	-66.74
Thiamine	1.30 mg	1.64	+26.15	1.58	+21.58	1.44	+10.77	1.66	+27.69	1.66	+27.31
Riboflavin	1.50 mg	0.66	-56.0	0.57	-62.00	0.56	-62.67	0.70	-53.33	0.68	-54.67
Niacin	16.00 mg	17.04	+6.50	17.37	+8.56	15.70	-1.88	18.22	+13.88	17.55	+9.70
Ascorbic acid	40.0 mg	61.03	+52.57	43.21	+8.03	57.20	+43.00	50.77	+26.93	51.79	+29.48

Source: Field Survey, 1999-2000.

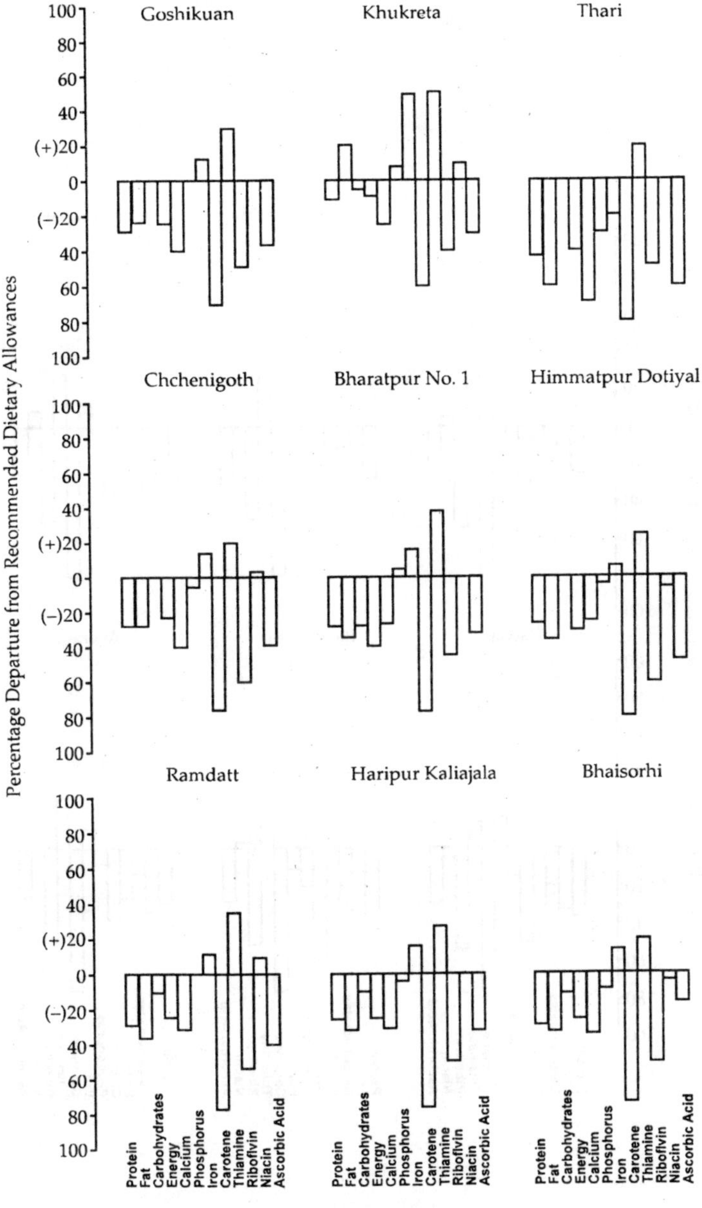

Fig. 5.6A. Nutrition Status of Lactating Category Women in the Sample Villages.

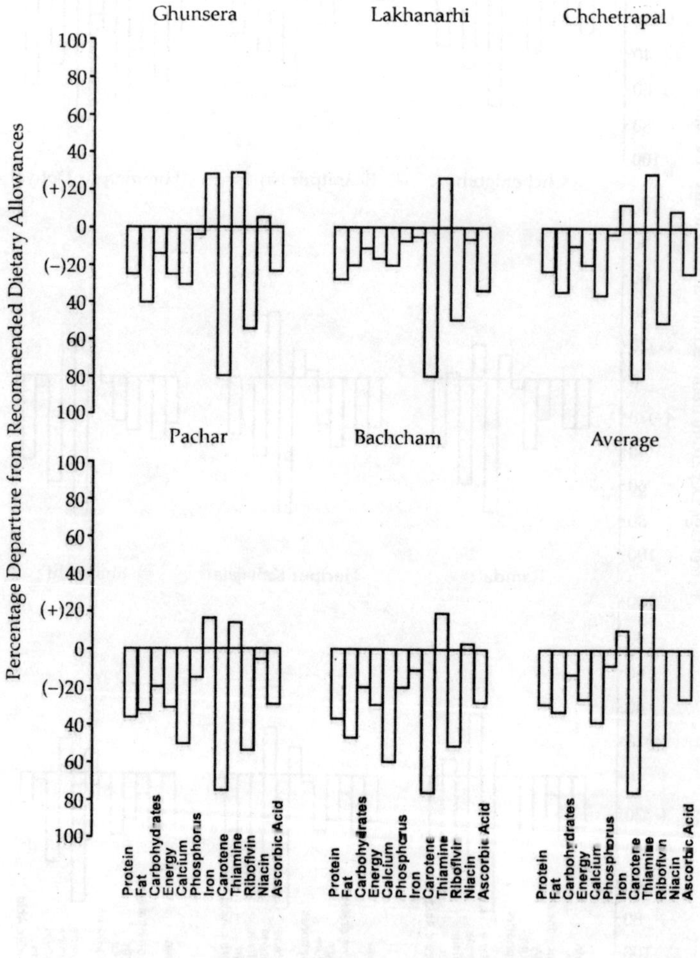

Fig. 5.6B: Nutrition Status of Lactating Category Women in the Sample Villages.

Table 5.32. Per Head Per Day Nutrients Intake Pattern of Lactating Category Women in the Sample Villages

Nutrients	*Recommended Dietary Awareness (RDA)*	*Goshikuan*		*Khukreta*		*Thari*		*Chchenigoth*		*Bharatpur No. 1*	
		Actual Intake	*Percentage Departure from RDA (+) (–)*	*Actual Intake*	*Percentage Departure from RDA (+) (–)*	*Actual Intake*	*Percentage Departure from RDA (+) (–)*	*Actual Intake*	*Percentage Departure from RDA (+) (–)*	*Actual Intake*	*Percentage Departure from RDA (+) (–)*
1	2	3	4	5	6	7	8	9	10	11	12
Protien	72.0 gm	51.13	-28.97	61.64	-14.39	40.96	-43.11	50.00	-30.55	53.15	-26.18
Fat	45.0 gm	32.57	-27.62	54.09	+20.20	18.11	-59.75	31.27	-30.51	32.25	-28.29
Carbohydrates	430.0 gm	365.86	-14.92	408.49	-5.00	336.26	-21.80	375.05	-12.78	312.64	-27.29
Energy	2700 K cal	1971.28	-26.99	2394.82	-11.30	1672.73	-38.05	2002.75	-25.82	1780.78	-34.05
Calcium	1000.0 mg	588.74	-41.13	752.05	-24.80	326.89	-67.31	595.05	-40.49	743.06	-25.69
Phosphorus	1400.00 mg	1408.14	+0.58	1582.78	+13.06	1010.88	-27.79	1305.26	-6.77	1503.51	+7.39
Iron	30.0 mg	35.01	+16.70	42.93	+43.10	26.29	-12.37	34.31	+14.37	35.86	+19.53
Carotene	3800.0 µg	882.13	-76.79	1452.38	-61.78	519.02	-86.34	843.85	-77.79	851.61	-77.59
Thiamine	1.35 mg	1.71	+26.67	1.99	+47.41	1.60	+18.52	1.66	+22.96	1.84	+36.30
Riboflavin	1.55 mg	0.80	-48.39	0.87	-43.87	0.76	-50.97	0.68	-56.13	0.84	-45.81
Niacin	17.5 mg	17.40	-0.57	19.18	+9.60	16.18	-7.54	17.77	+1.54	15.48	-11.54
Ascorbic acid	80.0 mg	53.42	-33.23	55.11	-31.11	30.98	-61.28	48.10	-39.80	53.34	-33.32

Contd.

Nutrients	Recommended Dietary Allowance (RDA)	Himmatpur Dotiyal		Ramdatt		Haripur Kaliajala		Bhaisorhi		Ghunsera	
		Actual Intake	Percentage Departure from RDA (+) (–)	Actual Intake	Percentage Departure from RDA (+) (–)	Actual Intake	Percentage Departure from RDA (+) (–)	Actual Intake	Percentage Departure from RDA (+) (–)	Actual Intake	Percentage Departure from RDA (+) (–)
1	2	13	14	15	16	17	18	19	20	21	22
Protien	72.0 gm	49.51	-31.24	52.64	-29.89	50.73	-29.54	46.07	-36.01	50.58	-29.75
Fat	45.0 gm	26.06	-42.09	27.53	-38.82	27.81	-38.20	27.42	-39.07	26.03	-42.16
Carbohydrates	430.0 gm	326.53	-24.06	384.05	-10.69	352.80	-17.95	345.41	-17.58	360.88	-16.07
Energy	2700.0 Kcal	1770.36	-34.43	2019.97	-25.19	1888.29	-30.06	1825.91	-32.37	1901.79	-29.56
Calcium	1000.0 mg	697.85	-30.22	658.91	-34.11	625.92	-37.41	606.61	-39.34	673.55	-32.65
Phosphorus	1400.00 mg	1356.81	-3.09	1401.74	+0.12	1336.86	-4.51	1236.96	-11.65	1357.83	-3.01
Iron	30.0 mg	31.04	+3.47	33.91	+13.03	36.16	+20.53	34.41	+14.70	37.60	+25.33
Carotene	3800.0 µg	698.61	-81.62	732.08	-80.73	740.13	-80.52	747.21	-80.34	694.73	-81.72
Thiamine	1.35 mg	1.66	+22.96	1.84	+36.30	1.75	+26.63	1.58	+17.04	1.72	+27.41
Riboflavin	1.55 mg	0.74	-52.26	0.74	-52.26	0.70	-54.84	0.62	-60.00	0.70	-54.84
Niacin	17.5 mg	16.33	-6.69	18.49	+5.66	17.40	-0.57	16.81	-3.94	17.85	+2.00
Ascorbic acid	80.0 mg	48.43	-39.09	52.29	-34.64	50.08	-37.4	67.09	-16.14	63.19	-21.01

Contd.

Nutrients	Recommended Dietary Allowance (RDA)	Lakhanarhi		Chchetrapal		Pachar		Bachcham		Average of the Sample	
		Actual Intake	Percentage Departure from RDA (+) (–)	Actual Intake	Percentage Departure from RDA (+) (–)	Actual Intake	Percentage Departure from RDA (+) (–)	Actual Intake	Percentage Departure from RDA (+) (–)	Actual Intake	Percentage Departure from RDA (+) (–)
1	2	23	24	25	26	27	28	29	30	31	32
Protien	72.0 gm	47.26	-34.36	52.41	-27.21	44.58	-38.08	43.29	-39.88	49.57	-31.16
Fat	45.0 gm	31.83	-29.27	28.82	-35.96	28.92	-35.73	21.94	-51.24	29.62	-34.18
Carbohydrates	430.0 gm	362.57	-15.68	393.42	-8.51	344.00	-20.00	349.20	-18.79	358.37	-16.66
Energy	2700.0 Kcal	1945.80	-27.93	2059.80	-23.71	1827.08	-32.33	1767.21	-34.55	1916.33	-29.02
Calcium	1000.0 mg	718.09	-28.19	598.45	-40.16	538.15	-46.19	362.57	-63.74	606.14	-39.39
Phosphorus	1400.00 mg	1295.78	-7.44	1395.12	-0.35	1173.87	-16.15	1138.65	-18.67	1321.73	-5.59
Iron	30.0 mg	28.17	-6.10	34.75	+15.83	34.57	+15.23	26.97	-10.10	33.71	+12.38
Carotene	3800.0 μg	837.56	-77.96	755.33	-80.12	784.81	-79.35	569.75	-85.01	793.51	-79.12
Thiamine	1.35 mg	1.67	+23.70	1.80	+33.33	1.54	+14.07	1.56	+15.56	1.71	+25.56
Riboflavin	1.55 mg	0.70	-54.84	0.72	-53.55	0.61	-60.65	0.56	-63.87	0.72	-53.73
Niacin	17.5 mg	16.48	-5.83	19.34	+10.51	16.37	-6.46	17.71	+1.20	17.34	-0.90
Ascorbic acid	80.0 mg	51.01	-36.24	58.81	-26.49	57.13	-28.59	49.95	-37.56	52.80	-34.00

Source: Field Survey, 1999-2000.

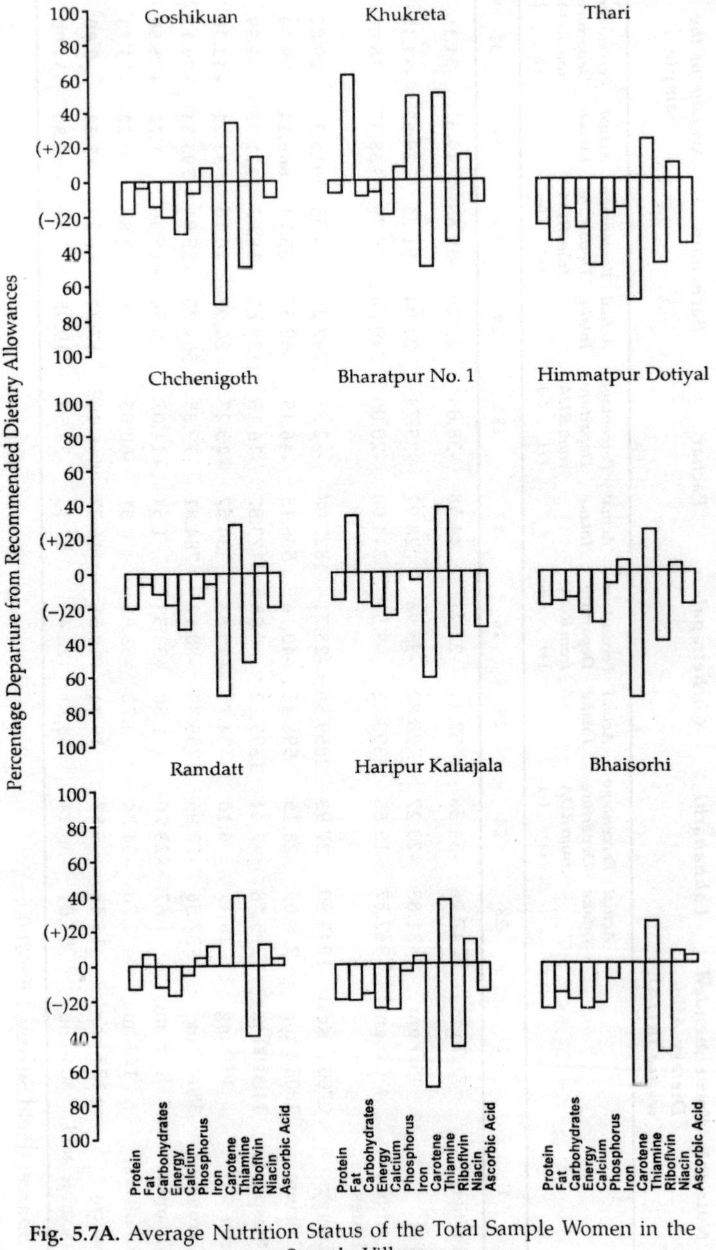

Fig. 5.7A. Average Nutrition Status of the Total Sample Women in the Sample Villages.

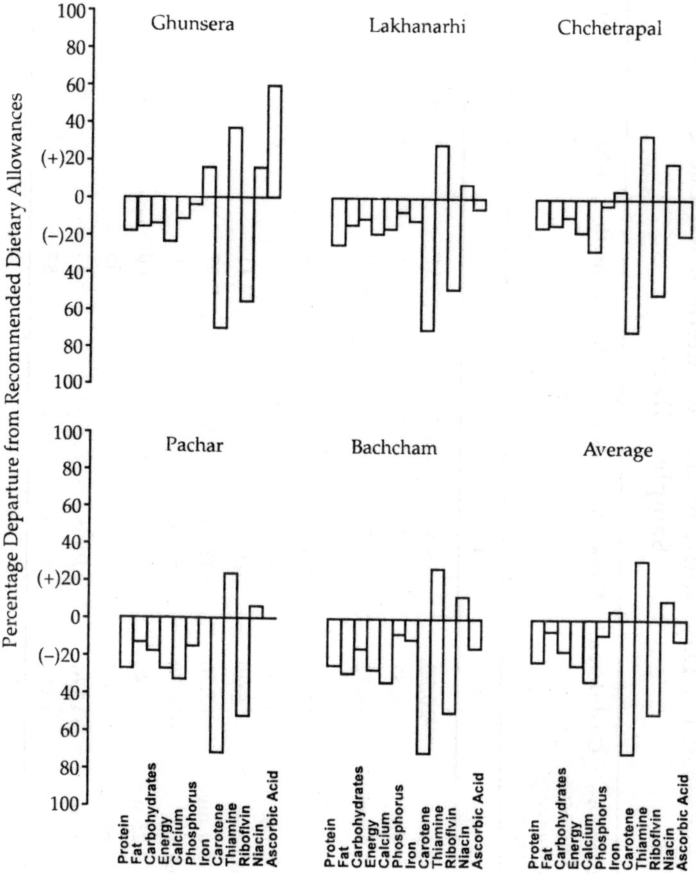

Fig. 5.7B. Average Nutrition Status of the Total Sample Women in the Sample Villages.

Table 5.33. Per Head Per Day Nutrients Intake Pattern of All Category Women in the Sample Villages

(Percentage Departure from the RDA)

Nutrients	*Recommended Dietary Allowance (RDA)*	*Goshikuan*	*Khukreta*	*Thari*	*Chchenigoth*	*Bharatpur No. 1*	*Himmatpur Dotiyal*	*Ramdatt*
1	2	3	4	5	6	7	8	9
Protein	62 gm	-20.58	-6.44	-29.77	-23.31	-16.90	-25.65	-12.76
Fat	32 gm	-3.53	+62.78	-35.78	-9.22	+30.50	-25.28	-5.38
Carbohy drates	130.0 gm	-16.12	-7.25	-19.31	-14.08	-17.75	-23.30	-12.25
Energy	2483 kcal	-22.03	-6.56	-29.63	-20.74	-18.76	-30.14	-16.99
Calcium	800 mg	-31.94	-19.13	-58.41	-33.05	-24.43	-33.82	-4.80
Phosphorus	1400 mg	-6.29	+9.64	-21.72	-17.41	-0.61	-11.25	+1.89
Iron	33.0 mg	+7.30	+43.82	-20.51	-7.27	-3.94	+4.36	+10.33
Carotene	2867 µg	-70.70	-51.80	-80.35	-73.16	-61.76	-77.63	-68.72
Thiomine	1.25 mg	+34.40	+55.20	+25.60	+29.60	+40.80	+27.20	+40.80
Riboflavin	1.68 mg	-52.41	-40.69	-57.24	-56.55	-31.03	-37.24	-40.69
Niacin	15.8 mg	+13.67	+19.68	+10.57	+9.43	+7.78	+3.86	+13.80
Ascorbic acid	60.0 mg	-10.98	-13.72	-45.40	-19.87	-26.27	-21.68	+1.45

Contd.

Nutrients	*Recommended Dietary Allowance (RDA)*	*Haripur kalia-jala*	*Bhaisorhi*	*Ghunsera*	*Lakhan-arhi*	*Chchetra-pal*	*Pachar*	*Bachc-ham*	*Total Average of the Sample*
1	2	10	11	12	13	14	15	16	17
Protein	62 gm	-18.39	-25.50	-18.66	-24.21	-16.61	-26.16	-23.90	-20.56
Fat	32 gm	-17.22	-14.75	-19.97	-14.28	-15.53	-13.50	-25.56	-6.48
Carbohy-drates	430.0 gm	-15.26	-20.51	-17.44	-11.68	-10.01	-17.35	-14.57	-15.49
Energy	2483 kcal	-22.74	-26.86	-21.85	-20.84	-18.80	-24.74	-24.74	-21.78
Calcium	800 mg	-23.96	-21.51	-12.56	-18.55	-25.61	-29.75	-39.98	-26.97
Phosphorus	1400 mg	-4.45	-11.93	-4.07	-9.20	-2.16	-12.82	-10.30	-7.19
Iron	33.0 mg	+1.12	-0.21	+15.73	-14.15	+1.48	-0.09	-13.21	+01.79
Carotene	2867 µg	-75.36	-74.44	-76.03	-74.32	-74.82	-74.28	-78.23	-72.26
Thiomine	1.25 mg	+37.60	+24.00	+36.80	+34.40	+40.80	+26.40	+31.20	+34.40
Riboflavin	1.68 mg	-52.41	-56.55	-51.72	-53.79	-51.03	-56.55	-56.55	-49.66
Niacin	15.8 mg	+13.04	+5.13	+14.43	+9.24	+18.35	+7.34	+14.81	+11.52
Ascorbic acid	60.0 mg	-12.65	+4.17	+60.75	-4.62	-15.83	-0.60	-15.43	-11.62

Source: Field Survey 1999-2000, and Gopalan, *et al.* 1993.

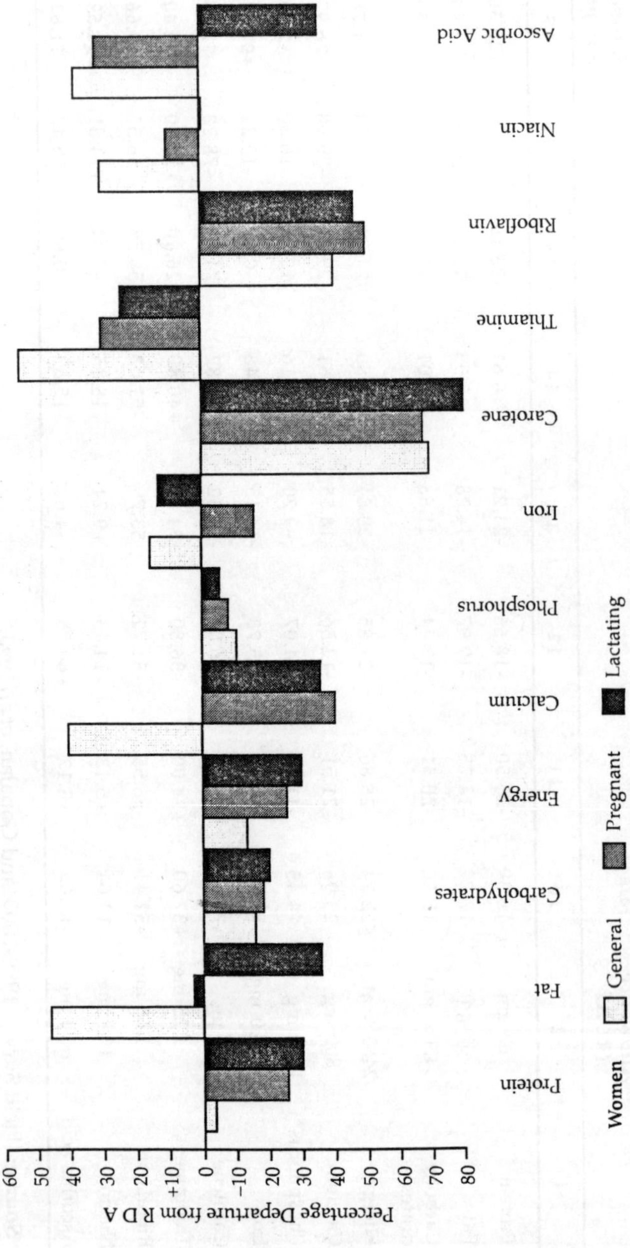

Fig. 5.8. Nutrition Status of the Sample Women.

mg in Ghunsera village. The per head per day intake of ascorbic acid was found 54.49 mg by general category women 51.79 mg by pregnant women which are 36.23 and 29.48% above the standard requirement while the ascorbic acid intake by lactating women was found 52.80 mg which is 34% below the standard requirement of 80 mg. Village and Categorywise consumption of ascorbic acid is presented in tables 5.30-5.33 and figures 5.4 to 5.7.

There are many other factors that also influence the diet requirement such as climate, age, sex, activity, physiological status, community etc. in the food and nutrients intake pattern much disparity was seen in the regional and category level.

5.13 Mal Nutrition

The nutrition deficiency disease may not essentially be due to lack of single nutrient. It may occur due to the lack of more than one nutrient in the diet taken by the people for a specified duration of the year. The deficiency of one and more nutrients may produce different diseases in accordance with varying degree of deficiency of nutrients, human resistance capacity, variable climatic conditions, various endemic relationships to mal nutrition and deficiency conditions, differences of food items from place to place and one season to another. Nutritional deficiency is one of the serious problems in the hilly region (Pant, 1994, 1998 Pant and Jalal, 1991a and 1991b Jalal *et al.* 2001). The deficiency restrains their physical growth and mental development and make them more susceptible to morbility and mortality due to infectious diseases.

In the present study an attempt has been made to asses, on the basis of field study, the nutritional status of the each category women of 14 selected villages of the Uttarakhand Himalaya. For measuring the nutritional status, 136 sample women have been surveyed for the general, pregnant and lactating categories of major communities of all the 14 villages.

Table 5.34. Body Mass Index of General Category Women (Chronic Energy Deficiency, CED)

(% of the total Sample)

Group/ Classification	*Sample Villages*							
	Goshikuan	*Khukreta*	*Thari*	*Chchenigoth*	*Baharatpur No. 1*	*Himmatpur Dotiyal*	*Ramdatt*	*Haripur Kaliajala*
1	2	3	4	5	6	7	8	9
< 16 CED Grade III	–	–	–	–	–	–	–	–
16.01 – 17.0 CED Grade II	01 (33.33)	01 (33.33)	02 (66.67)	–	–	–	–	01 (33.33)
17.01–18.50 CED Grade I	–	–	–	02 (66.67)	–	01 (33.33)	01 (33.33)	02 (66.67)
18.51–20.0 CED Low Weight Normal	01 (33.33)	–	–	01 (33.33)	–	02 (33.33)	–	–
20.01–25.0 Normal	01 (33.34)	02 (66.67)	01 (33.33)	–	02 (100.00)	–	02 (66.67)	–
25.01–30.0 Obese Grade I	–	–	–	–	–	–	–	–
>30.01 Obese Grade II	–	–	–	–	–	–	–	–
Total	**03 (100)**	**03 (100)**	**03 (100)**	**03 (100)**	**02 (100)**	**03 (100)**	**03 (100)**	**03 (100)**

Contd.

Group/ Classification	*Bhaisorhi*	*Ghunsera*	*Lakhanarhi*	*Chchetrapal*	*Pachar*	*Bachcham*	*Total Sample*
1	10	11	12	13	14	15	16
<16 CED Grade III	–	–	–	–	–	–	–
16.01–17.0 CED Grade II	–	01 (33.33)	–	–	–	–	06 (15.38)
17.01–18.50 CED Grade I	–	01 (33.33)	01 (50.00)	01 (50.00)	–	02 (66.67)	11 (28.21)
18.51–20.0 CED Low Weight Normal	03 (100.00)	01 (33.34)	–	–	01 (33.33)	–	09 (28.08)
20.01–25.0 Normal	–	–	01 (50.00)	01 (50.00)	021 (66.67)	01 (33.33)	13 (39.33)
25.01–30.0 Obese Grade I	–	–	–	–	–	–	–
>30.01 Obese Grade II	–	–	–	–	–	–	–
Total	**03 (100)**	**03 (100)**	**02 (100)**	**02 (100)**	**03 (100)**	**03 (100)**	**39 (100)**

Source: Field Survey, 1999-2000.

Body Mass Index was calculated using the formula weight (kg)/height^2(m). Body Mass Index has been calculated for each category women,. Then BMI has been classified in to seven groups: - (1) Below 16 – CED grade III Severe, (2) 16.01 – 17.0 CED grade II Mild, (3) 17.01 – 18.5 CED grade I Moderate, (4) 18.51 – 20 Low Weight Normal, (5) 20.01 – 25.0 Normal, (6) 25.01-30.0 Obese grade I and (7) Above 30.01, Obese grade II.

Using BMI <18.5 as the criteria (optimum) for Chronic Energy Deficiency (CED). About 43.59% of total general women were found suffer from various degree of CED. Among them 15.38% were found to suffer from CED grade II (16.01 – 17.0 CED mild) and 28.21% from CED grade I (17.01 to 18.5 moderate) form of mal nutrition (Fig. 5.8).

Out of the total surveyed general category women 23.08% were found in low weight normal category (18.51-20.0) while 33.33% were found in normal category (20.01-25.0). The mean BMI of general category women was 19.24. Villagewise BMI of general women is presents in table 5.34 and figure 5.8. Villagewise Body mass Index of pregnant women is presented in table 5.35 and figure 5.9. Table 5.36 shows that out of the total 44 samples about 36% were found suffer from the various degree of CED. Among them only one case (2.27%) was belongs to Bhaisorhi village was suffer from CED grade III (<16 CED, severe) while 9.1% were found suffer from CED grade II (mild). Out of the total 20.45% were found in CED low weight normal and 40.91% were in CED normal. Only one case (2.27%) resident of Chhetrapal village was found suffer from obese grade I (25.01-30.0). The mean BMI of pregnant women was 19.66. It is evident from table 5.43 that out of the total 53 lactating women about 47% women were found suffer from various degree of CED. Only one case (1.89%) was found suffer from CED grade I while 11.32% women were in the grade of CED II. Remaining 30.19 and 22.64% were found in low weight normal and normal category respectively. The mean BMI of the lactating women was 18.89 which is lower than the regional BMI of 19.26 (Table 5.36 and Figure 5.10).

Table 5.35. Body Mass Index of Pregnant Category Women (Chronic Energy Deficiency, CED)

(% of the total Sample)

	Sample Villages							
Group/ Classification	*Goshikuan*	*Khukreta*	*Thari*	*Chchenigoth*	*Baharatpur No. 1*	*Himmatpur Dotiyal*	*Ramdatt*	*Haripur Kaliajala*
1	2	3	4	5	6	7	8	9
< 16 CED Grade III	–	–	–	–	–	–	–	–
16.01 – 17.0 CED Grade II	–	–	01 (25.0)	01 (33.33)	–	02 (66.67)	–	–
17.01–18.50 CED Grade I	03 (100.00)	–	01 (25.0)	02 (66.67)	–	01 (33.33)	–	01 (33.33)
18.51–20.0 CED Low Weight Normal	–	–	01 (25.0)	–	–	–	01 (33.33)	01 (33.33)
20.01–25.0 Normal	–	03 (100.0)	01 (25.0)	–	02 (100.00)	–	02 (66.67)	01 (33.34)
25.01–30.0 Obese Grade I	–	–	–	–	–	–	–	–
>30.01 Obese Grade II	–	–	–	–	–	–	–	–
Total	**03 (100)**	**03 (100)**	**04 (100)**	**03 (100)**	**02 (100)**	**03 (100)**	**03 (100)**	**03 (100)**

Contd.

Group/ Classification	*Bhaisorhi*	*Ghunsera*	*Lakhanarhi*	*Chchetrapal*	*Pachar*	*Bachcham*	*Total Sample*
1	**10**	**11**	**12**	**13**	**14**	**15**	**16**
<16 CED Grade III	01 (33.33)	–	–	–	–	–	**01 (2.27)**
16.01–17.0 CED Grade II	–	–	–	–	–	–	**04 (9.10)**
17.01–18.50 CED Grade I	–	–	–	01 (33.33)	01 (25.00)	01 (25.00)	**11 (28.21)**
18.51–20.0 CED Low Weight Normal	–	01 (33.33)	02 (66.67)	01 (33.33)	01 (25.00)	01 (25.00)	**9 (20.45)**
20.01–25.0 Normal	02 (66.67)	02 (66.67)	01 (33.34)	–	02 (50.00)	02 (50.00)	**18 (40.9)**
25.01–30.0 Obese Grade I	–	–	–	01 (33.34)	–	–	**01 (2.27)**
>30.01 Obese Grade II	–	–	–	–	–	–	–
Total	**03 (100)**	**03 (100)**	**02 (100)**	**02 (100)**	**04 (100)**	**04 (100)**	**44 (100)**

Source: Field Survey, 1999-2000.

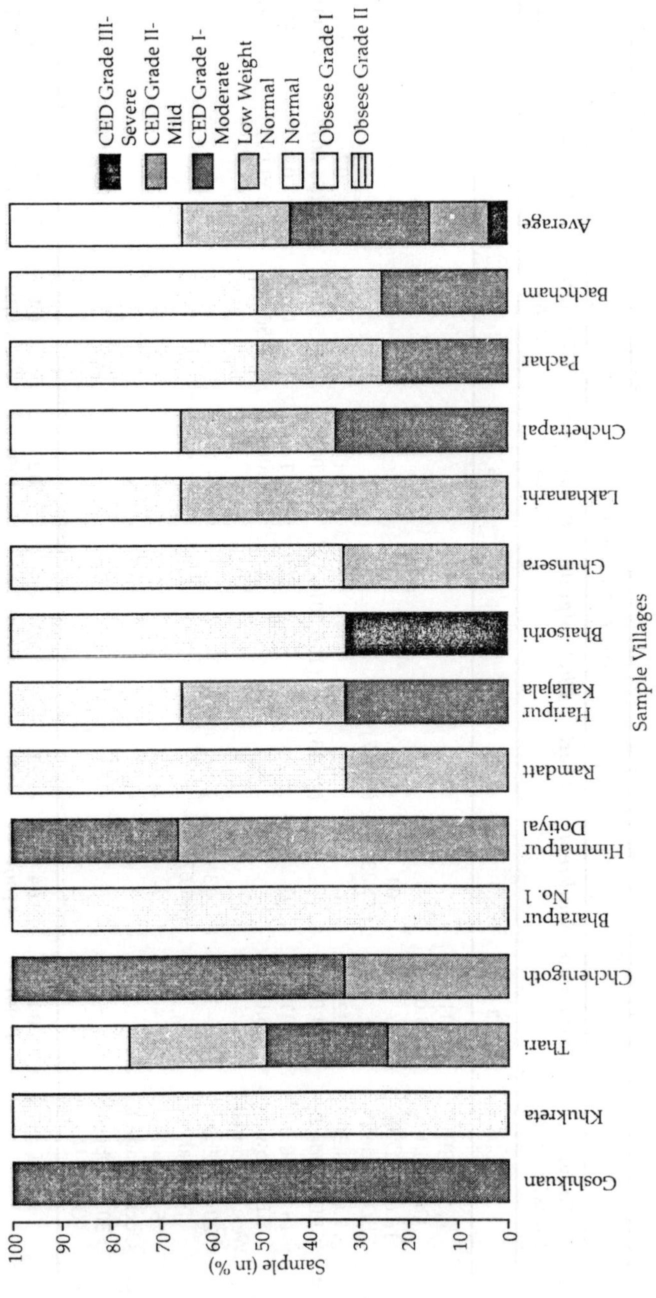

Fig. 5.9. Chronic Energy Deficiency (CED) in the General Category Women.

Table 5.35. Body Mass Index of Pregnant Category Women (Chronic Energy Deficiency, CED)

(% of the total Sample)

	Sample Villages							
Group/ Classification	*Goshikuan*	*Khukreta*	*Thari*	*Chchenigoth*	*Baharatpur No. 1*	*Himmatpur Dotiyal*	*Ramdatt*	*Haripur Kaliajala*
1	2	3	4	5	6	7	8	9
< 16 CED Grade III	01 (25.00)	–	–	–	–	–	–	–
16.01 – 17.0 CED Grade II	–	01 (33.33)	02 (66.67)	–	–	–	–	01 (25.00)
17.01–18.50 CED Grade I	02 (50.00)	–	01 (33.33)	04 (100.00)	01 (50.00)	02 (50.00)	02 (50.00)	02 (50.00)
18.51–20.0 CED Low Weight Normal	01 (25.00)	–	–	–	01 (50.00)	02 (50.00)	02 (50.00)	01 (25.00)
20.01–25.0 Normal	–	03 (66.67)	–	–	–	–	–	–
25.01–30.0 Obese Grade I	–	–	–	–	–	–	–	–
>30.01 Obese Grade II	–	–	–	–	–	–	–	–
Total	**04 (100)**	**04 (100)**	**03 (100)**	**04 (100)**	**02 (100)**	**04 (100)**	**04 (100)**	**04 (100)**

Contd.

Group/ Classification	*Bhaisorhi*	*Ghunsera*	*Lakhanarhi*	*Chchetrapal*	*Pachar*	*Bachcham*	*Total Sample*
1	10	11	12	13	14	15	16
<16 CED Grade III	–	–	–	–	–	–	01 (1.89)
16.01–17.0 CED Grade II	–	01 (25.00)	–	–	–	01 (33.33)	06 (11.32)
17.01–18.50 CED Grade I	02 (50.00)	–	01 (20.00)	01 (20.00)	–	–	18 (33.96)
18.51–20.0 CED Low Weight Normal	01 (25.00)	02 (50.00)	02 (40.00)	01 (20.00)	02 (66.67)	01 (33.33)	16 (33.96)
20.01–25.0 Normal	01 (25.00)	01 (25.00)	02 (40.00)	03 (60.00)	01 (33.33)	01 (33.33)	12 (22.64)
25.01–30.0 Obese Grade I	–	–	–	–	–	–	–
>30.01 Obese Grade II	–	–	–	–	–	–	–
Total	**04 (100)**	**04 (100)**	**05 (100)**	**05 (100)**	**03 (100)**	**03 (100)**	**53 (100)**

Source: Field Survey, 1999-2000.

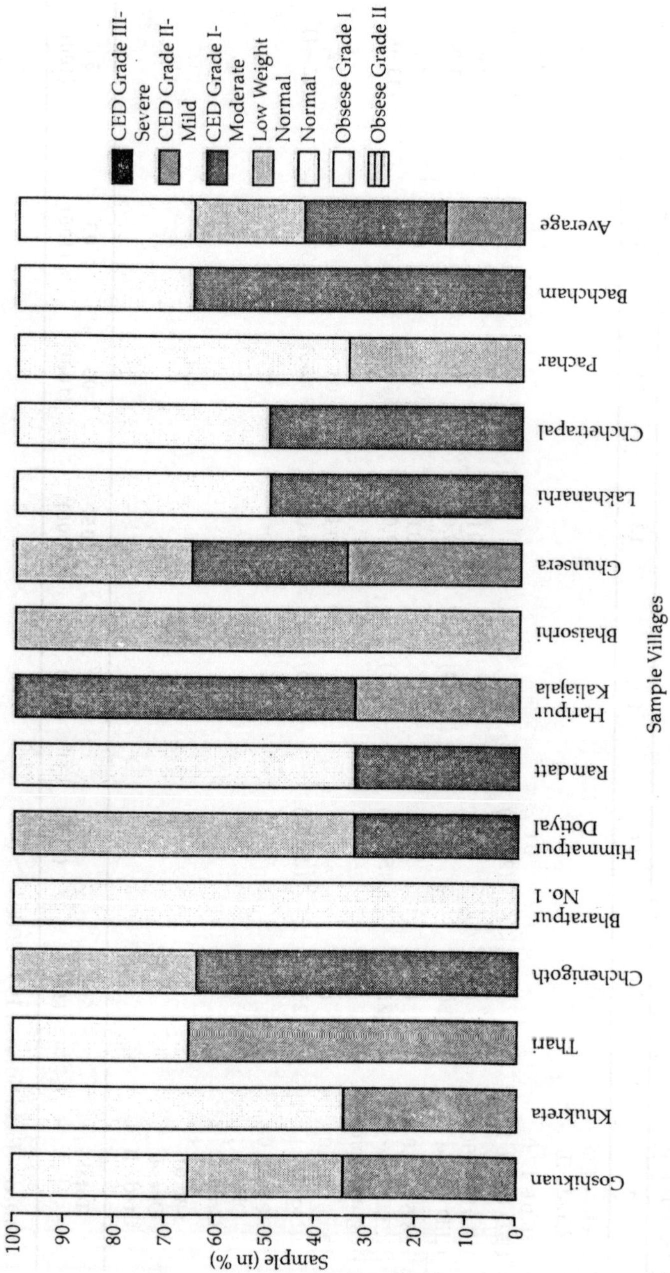

Fig. 5.10. Chronic Energy Deficiency (CED) in the Pregnant Category Women.

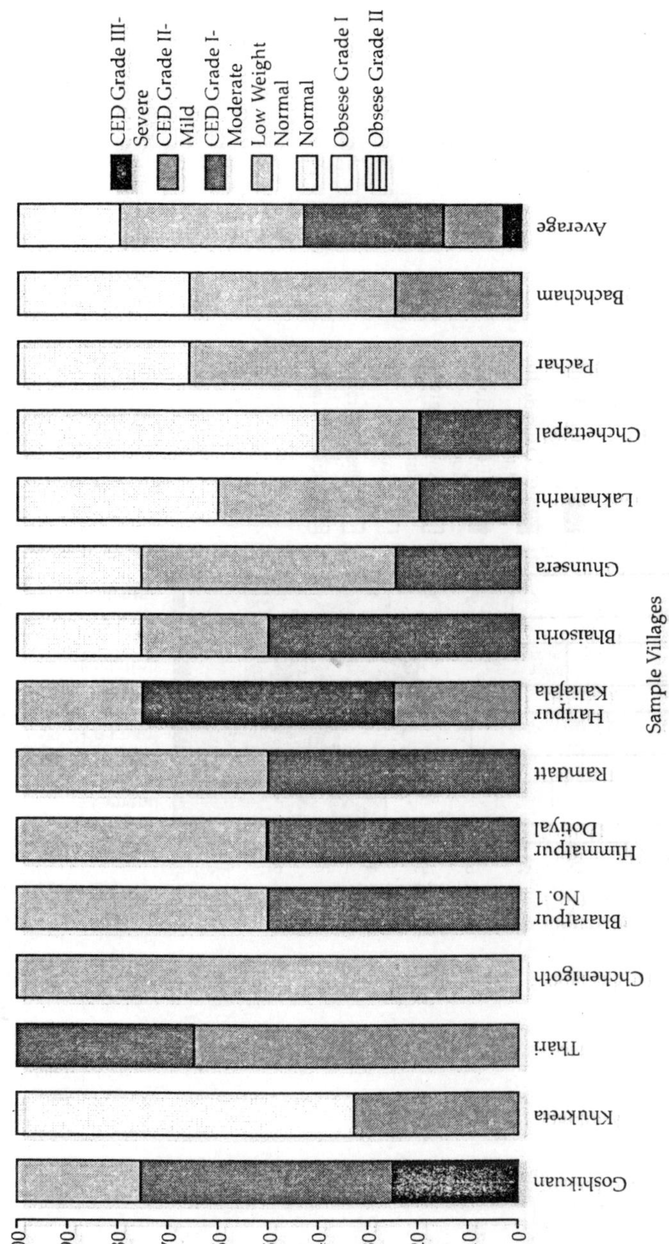

Fig. 5.11. Chronic Energy Deficiency (CED) in the Lactating Category Women.

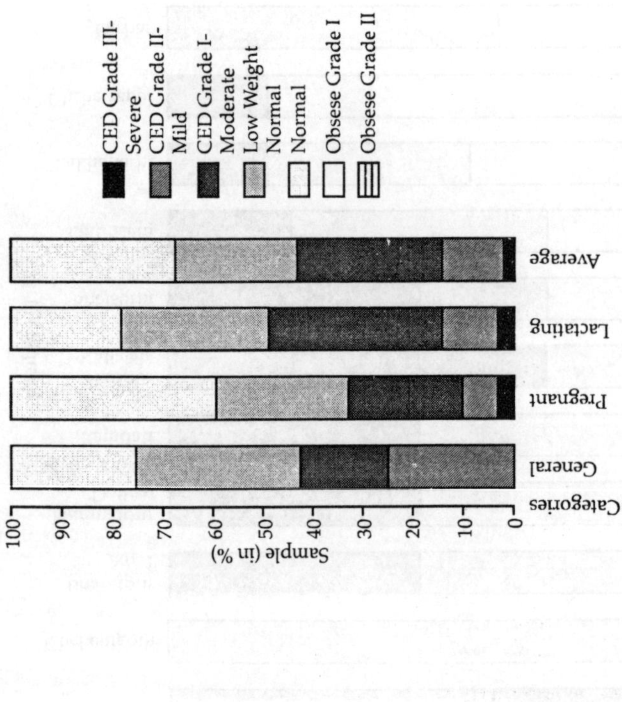

Fig. 5.12. Average Chronic Energy Deficiency (CED) in Total Sample Women.

A particular deficiency disease among the sample with the correlation of a particular deficiency of food nutrients has not been worked out in the present study. However number of studies done by the several authors in various part of the country indicates the close relationship between the nutrients intake and deficiency diseases.

5.14 Awareness Status

An attempt has been made here to find out the number of women who were aware about the mal nourishment (Table 5.44). In this regard majority (73.53%) of the total sample were not aware about mal nourishment. However, 70% of the total respondants told that they cooked their food item with cover. It also tried and find out that how many samples felt themselves physically good (fit) or bad (unfit). In this regard 70% samples were felt themselves physically fit or good while 30% were felt bad i.e. they were suffering from physical disorder. It was noticed, during the filed study that out of the total 136 sample 09 (6.62%) were found patient i.e. suffering from diseases. Treatment of four patients i.e. less than 50% were done by MBBS doctor while 2 were visited to Registered Medical Practitioner Clinic and one was treated by local vaidya. Remaining two were not visited anywhere (Table 5.37). Overwhelming proportion of the sample were not satisfied with medical facilities established nearby the villages. For any serious health problem they had to walk or traveled a long distances. Out of the total sample women 71.32% women were aware about the family planning but only 13.97% were adopted family planning measures (Table 5.38). A lot of misunderstandings about the family planning were prevalent among the samples.

Although the region is rich in medicinal plants and herbal which play an important role in the rural society. Numbers of plants are used in the daily life of the people. But 36.76 of the total sample were known about the important role of medicinal plants (Table 5.37). It is observed that old or any expert of the

Table 5.37. Awareness About Health Among the Sample

Particular	*Responses*	*Category of the Sample*			*Total*
		General	*Pregnant*	*Lactating*	
Cooking Pattern	Open	12 (69.23)	15 (34.09)	20 (37.74)	**47** **(34.56)**
	Covered	27 (30.77)	29 (65.91)	33 (62.26)	**89** **(65.44)**
Knowledge about mal nourishment	Yes	08 (20.51)	13 (29.55)	15 (28.30)	**36** **(26.47)**
	No	31 (79.49)	31 (70.45)	38 (71.70)	**100** **(73.53)**
Feeling about physical fitness	Good	22 (56.41)	20 (45.45)	30 (56.60)	**72** **(52.94)**
	Bad	17 (43.59)	24 (54.55)	23 (43.40)	**64** **(47.06)**
Patient (No.) (% of the total sample)	–	05 (12.85)	01 (2.27)	03 (5.66)	**09** **(6.62)**
Treatment by	RMP	01 (20.00)	– –	01 (33.33)	**02** **(22.22)**
	Vaidya	01 (20.00)	01 (100.00)	–	**01** **(11.11)**
	Doctor	03 (60.00)	–	01 (33.33)	**04** **(44.45)**
	No Treatment	Nil		01 (33.34)	**02** **(22.22)**
Knowledge about medicinal plants/herbs	Yes	14 (35.90)	18 (40.91)	18 (33.96)	**50** **(36.76)**
	No	25 (64.10)	26 (59.09)	35 (66.04)	**86** **(63.24)**

Source: Field Survey, 1999-2000.

Note: Figures are shown in parenthesis refer to the percentage of total sample in each category.

medicinal plants do not want to share this important information to their coming generations. They believed that the importance of the thing would be lost due to its knowledge distribution. This misunderstanding must be rootout from the society through the awareness compaign and knowledge must be served for the welfare of the society.

Table 5.38. Awareness About Family Planning Programme Among the Sample

Particular	*Responses*	*Category of the Sample*			*Total*
		General (39 No.)	*Pregnant (44 No.)*	*Lactating (53 No.)*	
Knowledge about family planning	Yes	32 (82.05)	28 (63.64)	37 (69.81)	**97 (71.32)**
	No	07 (17.95)	16 (36.36)	16 (30.19)	**39 (28.68)**
Any family planning measure adopted	Yes	08 (20.15)	04 (9.09)	07 (13.21)	**19 (13.97)**
	No	31 (79.49)	40 (90.91)	46 (86.79)	**117 (86.03)**

Source: Field Survey, 1999-2000.

Note: Figures shown in parentheses refer to the percentage of total.

6

SUMMARY AND CONCLUSION

The nutrition status of the people is an important indicator of the development of a country. Despite spectacular increase in foodgrains in recent decades the problem of chronic malnutrition continues to exist extensively, especially among children and women because they are caught in relentless sequence of ignorance, poverty, inadequate nutritious food intake and disease. Health is a state of complete physical, mental and social well-being and not merely an absence of disease or infirmity.

India has the highest number of women dying during pregnancy and childbirth. According to a report, 410 out of every one lakh just born babies in the country lose their mother during the delivery itself. More than 75% of the total population reside in the rural areas and slums in India. The economy of the rural people depend on agricultural practices which are mostly performed by the neglected and ignored section of the society i.e. women, who constitute nearly 50% of the total population. Likewise India, women of Uttarakhand Himalaya also perform primary activities and contribute a major share of family economy. In this part of Himalaya, excess workload coupled with inadequate intake of nutritious food have led normal to severe mal/under nutritional problem among the women. The main objective of this study is to calculate the nutrition status of most vulnerable section among the people-women as per their stage – general, pregnant, and lactating including their socio-economic background and awareness status.

Women not only in the Himalaya but also in the world as a whole have a lower status than men in the society. Due to various women's movements in recent past there has been a considerable increase in interest in the health and nutrition problem of women in the country.

A number of macro and micro level studies have been made in the field of health and nutrition and its related field in recent decades. The present investigation on women and nutrition has been particularly studied by the scientists of WHO, UNICEF, NIN, NNMB, NFHS, NFI, International Institute of Population Sciences, Department of Women and Child Development, Govt. of India etc. Few individual studies were also carried out in this field. But these studies are primarily confined to other than Himalayan Region. The present study is basically carried out geographical point of view in the 14-sample villages of Uttarakhand Himalaya.

The study of 136 sample women – 39 general, 44 pregnant and 53 lactating have been randomly selected from the 14 sample villages located in different geographical locations of Uttarakhand Himalaya. Data pertaining to socio-economic base, hygiene condition, environmental sanitation, housing pattern, food intake etc. of the sample women has been collected with the help of well structured questionnaires during door to door survey. Overall information of the region has been gathered from secondary sources. The analysis of nutritional data has been done on the basis of data, information and techniques published by NIN, Indian Council of Medical Research, Hyderabad (Gopalan *et al.* 1993).

The Indian Himalaya is facing a number of environmental hazards such as massive landslides, accelerating soil erosion reducing soil productivity, drying springs, frequent earthquakes and uncontrolled flood which are manifestations of ruthless deforestation, rapid growth of population, negligence of administration and unawareness of the society on environmental issues. The Himalaya falls in India encompasses an area of about 5, 17,733 km^2 i.e. 15.75% of the country land area with 4.03,11,039 persons in 2001 accounting for about 3.92% population of the country. According to the 2001 census, population wise Jammu and Kashmir stands the largest state in the Himalaya accounts 0.98% of the country's population and the smallest state in Sikkim with a population of 540493 persons which is 0.05% of the total country. It has registered 24.75% growth during the 1991 to 2001 which is higher than the country's average (21.34%). Among the Himalayan states, Nagaland registered maximum 64.41% growth during the decade of 1991 to 2001. The density of Himalaya is 78 persons/km^2 as against 62 persons/km^2 at 1991 census. The average sex ratio of the Himalaya is 933 males/ 1000 females in 2001 which is equal to national average (933). Maximum literacy is in Mizoram (88.49%) where 90.69% males and 86.13% females are literates which is quite higher than the national and regional averages. The Himalayan region has mostly rural population but steadily the developing towns are attracting large proportion of this rural population. Together all the states of the Himalaya only 19.99% population was urban in 1991 which was quite lower than that of the national average (25.72%). There is an urgent need to improve the education status of the people particularly females, which is too low in the Himalayan region. Any approach adopted for planning in this region must be consider the aspects of man and his environment.

The Uttarakhand Himalaya, the region under study include five latitudinal physiographic-geological zones viz. the Tarai – Bhabar, the Siwalik with dun, the Lesser Himalaya, the Great Himalaya and the Trans Himalaya. Similarly, the region is divided into five lithotectonic units separated by several thrusts and faults. The Uttarakhand Himalaya is drained by the head water of River Ganga. It includes three river systems the Yamuna, the Ganga and the Kali. The Tarai, Bhabar and low lying valleys below 800 m elevation have hot and humid climate. Between 800–1200 m elevation it becomes subtropical, then temperate, cool temperate, cold temperate and above 3000 m elevation it is almost alpine.

There are nine types of forests –tropical moist deciduous, tropical dry deciduous, sub–tropical pine, sub–tropical dry evergreen, Himalayan moist temperate, Himalayan dry temperate, sub-alpine, moist alpine and dry alpine shrubs as a whole. The soil survey of the study region as a whole has not been carried out so far.

According to the census of India 2001 Provisional Population Totals, the 70.35 lakh people of Uttarakhand live in 15,117 villages and 64 towns. The density of population in 2001 varies from 37 persons/km^2 in Uttarkashi district to 424 persons/km^2 in Dehradun district while it was in 1991 respectively 30 and 329 persons/km^2. Total population of Uttarakhand increased 18.72% during 1991-2001 compared to 21.45% as a whole country. Maximum (57.19%) villages have population less then 200 persons while only 0.07% villages have more then 5000 persons. The number of urban centers which were 18 in 1901, rose to 74 in 1991 where 21.70% of the total population is concentrated. The average male-female ratio in 1991 were 976 females/1000 males – 851 in Dehradun and 1128 in Almora districts. The number of females in the urban dominated districts are fewer than that of rural based districts. The age structure of the population is pyramidal. The Uttarakhand exhibits higher degree of literacy (73.81%) as compared to the country (65.38%) as a whole in 2001. Male (85.91%) and female (61.68%) literacy of the region is also high more than the country (male–75.85% and female– 54.16%). The working population, which was 45.61% in 1961, declined to 36.36% in 1991. Out of the total 66.93% workers were in primary sector lower than the country (67.53%) as a whole. Among the main workers 89.13% were engaged in cultivation in comparison to 38.72% in the country. The occupational classification of female workers region in the indicate that about 93.16, 1.52 and 5.32 per cent of them were engaged in primary, secondary and tertiary sectors respectively. About 16.7% and 3.54% of the population in Uttarakhand belong to Scheduled Castes and Scheduled Tribes. Among them 24.78 and 23.56 per cent were literate 1981. About 6.3% of the total population are ex-servicemen and 30,000 men are serving in the armed forces alone in the region.

The land-use statistics showed that out of the total reported area, 64% of land is under forest (under Forest Department), 5.62% cultivable waste, 0.14% under current fallow, 1.13% other fallow, 5.3% not suitable for cultivation, 2.44% land other than cultivation, 3.94% considered as permanent pasture and grazing land, 3.81% under trees, bushes, gardens excluding cultivation and 13.62% devoted for the cultivation during 1989-90. Paddy, madua, wheat and barley are the main crops of the region. The average holding size of the region is 0.94 ha. About 71% of the holdings with 28.1% of total cultivated area are marginal holdings i.e. below 01 ha. On an average only 0.09 ha land goes to the per head share of the cultivated land in the region. The population pressure on cultivated, forest and pasture lands is considerable high. Out of total 1,60,353 ha area is under tropical, subtropical and temperate fruits.

A number of institutions which provide maximum facilities to its inhabitants are the appropriate indicators to understand the socio-economic status of the region. Keeping in mind the ratio between the number of institutions established in the region and population, Uttarakhand does not present a picture of undeveloped region but if undulating typography a ground extent would be consider the real picture of the region would be clear. Due to difficult topography and lack of transport means one cannot get benefit from these available institutions. The overall development of the region is quite poor. The study shows that the fully hill districts are least developed even the index of development has registered negative growth. Most of the motor roads in the region are lying along the river valleys. After China and Pakistan aggressions, the transport network in the region has been accelerated and number of new roads have been constructed. However, the lot of villages are still inaccessible by motor vehicles.

Total 136 sample – 39 general, 44 pregnant and 53 lactating category women have been selected from 14 sample villages for detailed study. Out of total 136, 27.94% sample women belong to Brahmin, 26.47% Chhatriya, 12.5% Scheduled Castes, 10.29% Scheduled Tribes, 8.82% Punjabi, 1.47% Rastogi, 10.29% OBC's and 2.21% are Muslims. Only 2.2% women are less than 18 years of age and about 8% were in age group of 46–60 years. Maximum (90%) belong to the age group of 19 to 45 years. It indicates that still the marriage age of the girls prevails below 18 years in the rural area. Among the below 18 years sample women (03), one was pregnant and two were lactating during the field study. Out of total 31.6% households have high sex ratio while remaining 68.39% have low sex ratio. The prominent factor for the low sex ratio in this region are son preference, unequal treatment given to boys and girls, neglect of female infants, early marriage, death during pregnancy, bad treatment to women and hard work. On contrary this an average sex ratio in the fully hill districts of Uttarakhand is high because of the out migration of male population from the villages. About 51.47% sample women were illiterates and of the literates 45.5% were educated upto primary standard.

Agriculture is the basic source of livelihood of the majority of the population in Uttarakhand Himalaya. Total 98.52% sample women were engaged in agricultural activities including livestock rearing. Women participation in the region is found in almost all the rural occupations. Besides all household activities women role in agricultural operations is very significant and their contribution workout to more than three fourth of the labour required for agricultural and animal husbandary operations. Consequently the life of rural women in this region is one of the extreme drugery, misery and deprivation. Overwhelming operation about 72% of the total sample were spent 16-20 working hours a day. This overburdend work, in the absence of proper nutritious diet and health care is bound to create serious health repercussions both for the mother and child. Study shows that 7.35% households were depend on only agricultural activities, while

30.15% households were depend on cultivation, animal rearing, labouring and other activities. Taking all the sample women together 5.15, 26.47, 2.67, 16.18 and 23.53 per cent sample women were respectively in the group of very low income, low, moderate, and very high income group respectively. It reflects that maximum about 60% sample women were below the poverty line. In the study region fifty per cent sample women were self reliant and fifty per cent were depend on market or other sources.

About 28% of the total sample women were below 40 kg weight which can be termed as low weight from pregnancy point of view and 60% women weight were between 41-50 kg while 11.76% women were more than 51 kg weight. Average weight of the samples was 44.29 kg only. The study indicates that women's height between 140 to 145 cm were 7.35% which can be termed as short statured. About 55.15% women were between 151-155 cm heights. This study shows that the weight in reference to height of the sample women was very low which supports the hardworking of the hill women. Using Body Mass Index (BMI) < 18.5 as the criteria (optimum) for Chronic Energy Deficiency (CED) – 42.54% of the total sample women were found suffer from various degrees of CED. Among than 14.47% were found to suffer from CED grade III (Severe), 11.76% from CED grade II (mild) and 29.41% from CED grade I (moderate) form of malnutrition.

The mean age at the time of marriage in the Uttarakhand varied from one place to another. It was 15.53 years in the hill compared to 18.3 years in the country as a whole in 1981. Out of the total sample 15.44% women have no children while 8.82% have more than 6. It is noticed that the average spacing between the consecutive deliveries was less than 2 years. In this sample population total 37 cases (27.21%) experienced at least one abortion or miscarriage. It is due to early marriage of women and extremely hard life and harsh condition of work coupled with nutrition deficiency. That out of 44 pregnant women about 64% were not vaccinised. It is noticed that the percentage of women who were visited a health facility and those who were visited at home by the health workers (ANM) were very low. Likewise pregnant women, 60.38% of lactating women were also not vaccinised during their pregnancy period. All deliveries of the sample women were normal. Majority of the rural women were unaware of alternate services even the 90 tablets of iron and folic acid. Maximum (88.68%) deliveries were at home and conducted (75.45%) by untrained dais and mostly neighbourers and relatives. Such type of care at the time of birth has a major role to play in determining the survival of mother and offspring. About 66% new born babies were immunized regularly and remaining 44% were not visited the hospitals as well as not attended by a health worker. Out of the total new born babies (53) only 24.53% infants weight were more than 2.51 kg i.e. optimum weight while 75.47% infants were below 2.5 kg weight. The main causes of low birth weight were poor calorie and protein intake by mothers during the pregnancy in one hand and hard work in difficult terrain on the other.

The health status of the people in any region largely depends upon the physical quality of the environment. Health is a crucial attribute of human resource and a healthy human population is the most – desired national assest. The condition of housing and environmental sanitation is very unhygienic in the sample villages as a whole without any differences between caste, classes and region. The waste water has been disposed off in open spaces by the majority (95.6%) of the households. Very few households (4.4%) have hygienic method of water disposal through covered drains. The situation of refused disposal is still worse as large majority of the households (84.6%) dumped their refuse in the open space. Not a single households used a covered ditch for this purpose. Furthermore, as only 11.8% of the households availed of toilet facilities while the large majority of the households used fields for defecation. The rural villages of this region require a thorough management of water supply and sanitation with intensive awareness compaign. The infrastructural point of view the sample villages are very undeveloped.

Out of the total sample surveyed 41.18% brush their teeth and 30.88% women took bath daily. About 80.88% women were washed their hands before taking meal and 93% of the sample women have absence of hygienic sense.

The dietary habits of the region depends mostly upon the production of the particular areas. Generally the women of the sample villages took their food three times (53.68%) in a gastronomic day. Of total 39.71% women were regularly taking fast (upwas) a particular day in a week. Heavy work load couple with fast affect their health adversely. About 20% samples were bidi and tobacco is smokers while 2.94% both were bidi and tobacco smokers and country made liquor drinkers. Taking liquor, bidi and tobacco is not only affects the mother's health but also injurious for their offspring's health. It is find out that 49.26, 27.97 and 15.44 per cent women have took milk, curd and ghee daily while 22.06, 21.33 and 22.06 percent women did not consumed respectively these items even occasionally. Likewise daily pulse intake accounts for only 5.15% of the total sample while 93.32% women have consumed green vegetables monthly.

About 61.65% samples were non-vegetarian but 16.30% were consumed these products weekly. Some of the vegetables like brinjal, pumpkin, cauliflower, palak (Spinach) etc. even fruits were prohibited for lactating women in the sample villages. The diet of the study region is primarily based on cereals. On an average per capita per day cereal intake was 389.29 grams which is 11.53% less than the standard requirement of 440 grams, 50% villages were found less than the regional average. The cereal intake of all category women were also less than the normal requirement. Per capita daily intake of pulses was only 23.18 grams which is 48.49% less than the standard requirement of 45 grams. It varied in the villages from minimum 15.1 grams to maximum 46.6 grams. The per capita daily consumption of vegetables, cooking oil, sweet, milk products and fruits were less than the standard requirement. From the edible items consumption point of view there were no much more difference between the general, pregnant and lactating women. It is observed that its inhabitants particularly women were not aware about the essential intake of other food items such as pulses, vegetables, fruits etc even during the pregnancy and lactating periods. Because of this they consumed more cereals than other items.

Out of total energy intake 70-80% is drawn from cereals. In all, the average energy intake per capita per day was found 1942.2 kcal which is 21.78% below the standard requirement of 2483 kcal. The per head energy intake of general category women was found 1957.99 kcal which is 12% below the normal requirement of 2225 kcal. Similarly per capita daily energy intake of pregnant and lactating women was 23.09% and 29.02% below the standard requirement of 2525 kcal and 2700 kcal respectively. Almost 71% of the total sample village, the consumption of energy intake was found less than 2000 kcal. The average per capita per day protein intake was found 49.25 grams which is 20.56% below the standard requirement of 62 grams. Similarly the protein intake was found 1.16, 24.97 and 30.96 per cent less than the standard requirement among general, pregnant and lactating women respectively. The average fat intake per capita per day was found 29.81 grams which is 6.48% below the standard requirement of 32 grams. The per head daily fat intake by general category women was found 29.46 grams while 30.11 and 29.62 grams intake by pregnant and lactating women respectively which are 48.58% and 0.03% more and 30.96% less than the standard requirement of 20, 30 and 45 grams respectively.

In the study region, average carbohydrates intake was found 363.37 grams per head per day which is 15.5% below the standard requirement of 430 grams. The per head daily consumption of carbohydrates by general women was found 370.01 grams, by pregnant women was 363.69 and 358.37 grams by lactating women which are 13.95, 15.42 and 16.6 per cent below the standard requirements. The average per capita daily calcium intake was found 544.52 mg in the region, which is 31.94% below the standard requirement of 800 mg. The average per head per day calcium intake of general category was found 40.61% above from the standard requirement of 400 mg while 41.57 and 39.36 per cent below calcium intake was noticed in pregnant and lactating category women respectively from the standard requirement of 1000 mg.

In the sample villages the average iron intake per capita per day was found 33.59 mg which is 1.79% above the standard requirements of 33 mg. The average per head per day iron intake of general and lactating category women was found respectively 20 and 12.37 per cent above the standard requirement of 30 mg while the daily iron intake in pregnant category women was found 13.95% below from the standard requirement of 38 mg. The per head per day phosphorous intake in all categories found below the standard requirements. In the study region the carotene (vitamin A) intake is unsatisfactory because the consumption of per capita per day in all categories was found below the standard requirement. The thiamine (vitamin B_1) intake in average was 1.68 mg per head per day which is 34.4% above the standard requirement of 1.25 mg. In all the categories of the sample villages, the daily consumption of thiamine was found above the standard requirement. The average riboflavin (vitamin B_2) intake was 0.68 mg per capita daily which is 53.10% below the standard requirement of 1.45 mg. The per head / day intake of riboflavin in general category was 0.79 mg, in pregnant 0.68 mg, and 0.72 mg intake was found in lactating category women which is respectively 39.23, 54.67 and 3.55 per cent below the standard requirement of 1.3, 1.5 and 1.55 mg. In the sample villages, the average niacin intake was found 17.62 mg which is 11.52% above the standard requirement of 15.8 mg. On an average all the sample villages of the region, the consumption of niacin was found above the standard requirement. Although the per head per day intake by lactating women was found only 0.91% below the standard. In the study region, the average intake of vitamin C was found 53.03 mg which is 11.62% fall short from the standard requirement of 60 mg. The per capita daily intake of ascorbic acid was found 54.49 mg by general category women and 51.79 mg by pregnant women which are 36.23 and 29.48 per cent above the standard requirment while the ascorbic acid intake by lactating women was found 52.80 mg which is 34% below the standard requirement. There are many other factors that also influence the diet requirement such as climate, age, sex, activity, physiological status, community traditions etc. In the food and nutrients intake pattern much disparity was seen in the regional and category level.

The nutrition deficiency may not essentially be due to lack of single nutrients. It may occur due to the lack of more than one nutrient in the diet taken by people. Nutritional deficiency is one of the serious problem in the hill region. The deficiency restrains their physical growth and mental development and make them more susceptible to morbidity and mortality. For measuring the malnutritional status, Body Mass Index (BMI) has been calculated for each category women and grouped into seven classes/levels/grades. Using BMI<18.5 as the criteria (optimum) for Chronic Deficiency Energy (CED), about 43.59% of total general category surveyed women were found suffer from various degree of CED. Among them 15.38% were found to suffer from CED grade II (mild) and 28.21% from CED grade I (moderate) form of malnutrition. Out of total surveyed general category women 23.08% were found in low weight normal category while 33.33% were found in normal category. The mean BMI of general category was 19.24. Out of total 44 pregnant category women, about 36% were found suffer from the various degree of CED. Among them only one case (2.27%) was suffering from CED grade III (severe) while 9.1% were found suffer from CED grade II (mild). Out of total 20.45% were found in CED low weight normal and 40.91% were in CED normal. Only one case (2.27%) was found suffer from obese grade I. The mean BMI of pregnant women was 19.66. Out of the total 53 lactating women about 47% women were found suffers from various degree of CED. Only one case (1.89%) was found suffer from CED grade III while 11.32% women were in grade of CED II. Remaining 30.19 and 22.64 per cent were found in low weight normal and normal category respectively. The mean BMI of the lactating women was 18.89 which is lower than the regional BMI of 19.26. A particular deficiency disease among the sample with the correlation of a particular deficiency of food nutrients has not been workout in the present study.

Majority (73.53%) of the sample selected in the villages were not aware about malnourishment. In overall sample women were not also aware about the health, hygiene, sanitation, food intake, medicare point of view. Due to the ignorance of these aspects they were suffering a lot of problems.

The study concluded that the major determinants of nutrition status of women are the education, income and awareness level towards health. To overcome mal and under nutritional problem following remedial measures – policy and programmes should be implemented.

- Implementation of compulsory schooling of girls up to the age of 14.
- Implementation of minimum age at Marriage Act of 18 for girls.
- Monitor immunizations programme.
- Supplementary feeding programme.
- Increase the health and medical facilities.
- Adult Education Programme.
- Organise maternal and child health care programmes.
- Innovative programme to provide income generating activities.
- Compaign on the equality of sexes (daughter and sons).
- Social movements for health, hygiene, sanitation, dietary habits, nutritional value of local produces, family planning, child bearing and rearing etc.
- Change in cropping pattern according to nutrients requirements and modification in food habits.
- Participation of women must be compulsory in all activities particularly in village development.
- Urgent need of thorough management of housing, water supply and sanitation.
- Knowledge about the use of medicinal plants and herbs should be provided and preserved.

References

Abbas, N. and V. Subramanian, (1984), "Erosion and Sediment Transport in the Ganga River Basin", *Indian Journal of Hydrology*, 69:173-182.

Agrawal, Anil, (1982), *The State of India's Environment, 1982,* A Citizens Report, Centre for Science and Environment, New Delhi.

Anonymous, (1953), *Reports of Experts Committee on Environmental Sanitation,* World Health Organization, Geneva.

Anonymous, (1980), National Nutrition Monitoring Bureau, *Annual Report 1974-79,* World National Institute of Nutrition, ICMR, Hyderabad.

Anonymous, (1981a), *Census of India,* U.P. series 22, Part Iia Primary Census Abstract.

Anonymous, (1981b), *Census of India,* U.P. series 22, Part Iib(ii) General Economic Tables.

Anonymous, (1982), *Report of the Task Force for the Study of Eco-development in the Himalayan Region,* Planning Commission, Govt. of India, New Delhi.

Anonymous, (1988), *Women in India, A Statistical Profile,* Department of Women and Child Development, Ministry of Human Resource Development, Govt. of India, New Delhi.

Anonymous, (1991a), *Census of India,* Primary Census Abstract GISNIC, Nainital.

Anonymous, (1991b), *Census of India,* Series I, India Paper 2 of 1991, Provisional Population Totals, Rural Urban Distribution.

Anonymous, (1992a), *Agricultural Statistics of Uttar Pradesh 1989-90,* Director, Agriculture Statistics and Crop Insurance, U.P., Krishi Bhawan, Lucknow.

Anonymous, (1992b), Planning Commission, *Eight Five Year Plan (1992-1997),* Govt. of India, New Delhi.

Anonymous, (1993a), *Statistical Diary,* Uttaranchal, U.P. Uttaranchal Department, State Planning Institute Lucknow, U.P.

Anonymous, (1993b), *Surface Water Drainage for Low-Income Communities,* World Health Organisation, Geneva.

Anonymous, (1998), *World Health Report 1997,* World Health Organisation, Reprinted by Bookwell, New Delhi.

Anonymous, (1999), *Statistical Diary,* State Planning Institute, Srinagar-Garhwal.

Anonymous, (2001), *Census of India,* 2001 Series I, Provisional Population Totals, Papers of 2001 supplement district totals.

Ashish, M., (1979), "Agricultural Economy of Kumaun Hills: Threat of Ecological Disaster," *Economic and Political Weekly,* June 23.

Bahuguna, S.L., (1981), "Science and Rural Development in Hill Region," In J.S. Singh, S.P. Singh and C. Shastri (eds.), *Science and Rural Development in Mountains,* Gyanodaya Prakashan, Nainital, 9-15.

Baird, D., (1947), *Social Class and Foetal Mortality,* Lancet ii : 531-535.

Bakar, N.R. H.J. Abu., (1996), *Working Women and Their Families: A Case Study,* Asian Profile 24(2): 131-141.

Banerji, D., (1985), *Health and Family Planning Service in India: An Epidemiological, Socio-Cultural and Poltical Analysis and a Perspectives,* Lok Prakash, New Delhi.

Barros, F.C., C.G. Vicoria, J.P., Vaughar and H.J. Estanislau, (1987), Perinatal Mortality in Southern Brazil : A Population Based Study of 7392 Birth, *Bulletin of World Health,* 65: 95-204.

Bhasin, V., (1990), *Habitat, Habitation and Health in the Himalayas,* Kanila Raj Enterprises, Delhi.

Bora, R.S., (2000), "Out-Migration: Some Policy Implications for Uttarakhand," In M.C. Sati and S.P. Sati (eds.), *Uttarakhand Statehood : Dimensions of Development,* Indus Public Co., New Delhi, 91-114.

Burrerd, S.G., H.H. Hayden and A.M. Hirons, (1933), *A Sketch of Geology and Geography of the Himalaya Mountain and Tibet,* Pt. 1:5.

Champion, H.G., and S.K. Seth, (1968), *A Revised Survey of the Forest Types of India,* Manager of Publications, Delhi.

Chatterjee, M., (1989), "Socio-Economic and Socio-Cultural Influences on Women's Nutritional Status and Roles," In C. Gopalan and S. Kaur (eds.), *Women and Nutrition in India,* NFI Special Publication, Series 5 : 296-323.

Chatterjee, M. and J. Lambert, (1990), "Women and Nutrition, Reflections from India and Pakistan," Acc/CAN Sysposition Report, *Nutrition Policy Discussion Paper No. 6,* Geneva, Administrative Committee on Coordination/Subcommittee on Nutrition, 73-108

Chaudhaury, F.I. and Frank Trovato, (1994), "The Role and Status of 'Women the Timing of Marriage' in 5 Asian Countries," *Journal of Comparative Family Studies,* 25 : 143-157.

Dhar, T.N., (1996), "Health and Human Development in Uttarakhand", in K.S. Valdiya (ed.), *Uttarakhand Today,* Shree Almora Book Depot, Almora, 127-132.

Dhar, T.N., and S.P. Gupta (1992), *The Himalayan States of India; Development Profile,* SHERPA, Lucknow, p. 408.

Geervani, P., P. Anuradha, P. Geetha Salaja, R. Sandhya Kumari and G. Nageshwar Rao, (1983), "The Consequences of Development Progrommes on the Nutrient Intake and Nutritional Status of Vulnerable Segments of Population in Andhra Pradesh," *Journal of National Institute of Rural Development,* 2(6) : 571-580.

Ghildyal, B.P., (1981), "Soils of the Garhwal and Kumaun Himalaya," In J.S. Lall and A.D. Moddie (eds.), *The Himalaya: Aspects of Change,* OUP, New Delhi, 120-137.

Gopalan, C., (1989a), *Nutrition, Health and National Development,* Nutrition Foundation of India Special Publication Series, p. 4:136.

Gopalan, C., (1989b), "Women and Nutrition in India–General Consideration," In C. Gopalan and S. Kaur (eds.), *Women and Nutrition in India,* NFI Special Publication, Series 5: 1-16.

Gopalan, C., B.V. Ramashastri and S.C. Balasubramanian Revised and Updated by B.S. Narsinga Rao, Y.G. Deosthale and K.C. Pant, (1993), *Nutritive Value of Indian Foods,* NIN, ICMR, Hyderabad, p. 156.

Gopalan, C., and Harvinder Kaur, (1993), *Towards Better Nutrtion, Problems and Policies,* NFI Special Publication Series, 9: p. 447.

Gopalan, C., and S. Kaur, (1989), (eds.) *Women and Nutrition in India,* NFI Special Publication, Series 5: p. 378.

Haigh, M.J., (1984), "Landslide Predication and Highway Maintenance," In the Lesser Himalaya, India, *Z. geomoph N.F. SB,* 51-17-38.

Haigh, M.J. J.S. Rawat and S.K. Bartarya, (1989), "Environmental Indicators of Landslide Activity Along the Kilbury Road Nainital," *Kumaun Himalaya Mountain Research and Development,* 9(1): 25-33.

Hazra, Jayati, (1998), Women and Health, *Geographical Review of India,* 60 (4): 518-533.

Ives, J.D. and B. Messerli, (1989), *The Himalayan Dilemma: Reconciling Development and Conservation,* The United Nations University Routledge, New York, p. 295.

Jalal, D.S., B.R. Pant and R.C. Joshi, (2001), *Environmental Study in Himalayan Region,* Anmol Publications Pvt. Ltd., New Delhi, p. 239.

James, W.P.T., L. Anna Ferro and J.C. Waterlow, (1988), "Definition of Chronic Energy Deficiency in Adults," European, *Journal of Clinical Nutrition,* 42: 969.

Jhingran, A.G., (1981), "Geology of the Himalaya," In J.S. Lall and A.D. Moddie (eds.), *The Himalaya: Aspects of Change,* Oxford University Press, New Delhi, 77-98.

Jhonstone, R.J., (1994), *Ed. Dictionary of Human Geography,* Blackwell Oxford, U.K., p. 242.

Joshi, A., P.S. Garia, and I. Hasnain, (1999), *Uttarakhand Update: A Statistical Profile for Development Planning,* Kanishka Publishers, Distributors, New Delhi, 404p.

Kanitkar, T., and K. Srinivasan, (1989a), "Demographic Cosequences of Low Status of Women in Indian Society," In C. Gopalan and S. Kaur (eds.), *Women and Nutrition in India,* N.F.I. Special Publication, Series 5: 17-62.

Karmarkar, T.D., V. Sampathkumar, S. Jeyalakshmi and R. Abel, (1995), "Nutritional Status of Tribal Women in Bihar," *Man in India,* 75(2): 209-214.

Kisanga, P., (1990), *Women and Nutrition,* Tanzania Food and Nutrition Centre Efforts in Improving the Nutrition of Women in Tanzania, ACC/SCN Symposium Report, Nutrition Policy Discussion, Paper No. 6: 133-143.

Kramer, M.S., (1987), "Determinants of Low Birth Weight," Methodological Assessment and Meta-Analysis, *Bull World Health,* 65 : 663-737.

Krasovec, L., (1991), "Pregnancy Weight, Background Issues," In K. Krasovec, M.A. Anderson (eds.), *Maternal Nutrition and Pregnancy Outcomes, Anthropometric Assessment,* Scientific Publication, No. 529, Pan American Health Organisation.

Mathai, S.T., (1989), "Women and the Health System," In C. Gopalan and S. Kaur (eds.), *Women and Nutrition in India,* NFI Special Publication, Series 5: 247-295.

Menard, H.W., (1963), *Some Rates of Regional Erosion,* Journal Geology, 69 : 154-161.

Pant, B.R., (1988), *Land Utilization in Kotadun, Kumaun Himalaya,* Ph.D. Thesis, Kumaun University, Nainital, p. 270.

Pant, B.R., (1992a), "An Appraisal of Land and Other Resources in Himalaya : A Case Study," *Indian Journal of Landscape Systems and Ecological Studies,* 15(2): 13-21.

Pant, B.R., (1992b), *An Appraisal of Health and Nutrition Status in Kumaun Himalaya,* Progress Report Submitted to the CSIR, New Delhi, 50 p (Memio).

Pant, B.R., (1994), *Food and Nutrition: A Study of Himalayan Region,* Anmol Publications, New Delhi, 195.

Pant, BR., (1995a), *The Central Himalaya: Geographical Outlook,* In B.R. Pant and M.C. Pant (eds.), *Glimpses of Central Himalaya: A Socio-Economic and Ecological Perspective,* Radha Publications, New Delhi, Pt. 1:3-86.

Pant, B.R., (1995b), "Nutrition Availability Pattern of Scheduled Tribe Population in Uttarakhand-Buksha A Case," *Geog. Review of India,* 54(4) : 358-366.

Pant, B.R., (1995c), "Food and Nutrition Intake Scenario of Tharu Tribes in Uttarakhand Himalaya," *Indian Journal of Landscape System and Ecological Studies,* 19(1) : 112-119.

Pant, B.R., (1996a), "Physical Geography and Demographic Structure of Uttarakhand," In K.S. Valdiya (ed.), *Uttarakhand Today,* Shree Almora Book Depot, Almora : 45-65.

Pant, B.R., (1996c), "A Geographical Study of Scheduled Castes Population in Uttarakhand (India)," *The Indonesian Journal of Geography,* 28(7) : 25-38.

Pant, B.R., (1998), *Geo-Economic Environment and Nutrition,* Anmol Publications Pvt. Ltd., New Delhi : 173p.

Pant, B.R., (2000a), *Uttarakhand : Demographic Scenario,* Uttara, 11(1) : 6-9.

Pant, B.R., (2000b), "Geographical Personality of Uttarakhand," In M.C. Sati and S.P. Sati (eds.), *Uttarakhand Statehood: Dimensions of Development,* Indus Pub. Co., New Delhi, 19-55.

Pant, B.R., (2001), *Women and Nutrition in Himalaya,* MRP Report submitted to the U.G.C. New Delhi, 136p (Memio).

Pant, B.R., (2002), "Drudgary and Nutrition Status of the Rural Women" in the Central Himalayas, *The Indonesian Journal of Geography,* Yogakarat, Indonesia, 34(1&2): 1-16.

Pant, B.R., (in Press, a), "Women and Nutrition in Himalayan Region: Uttarakhand," A case, *The Geographer.*

Pant, B.R., (2003), "Mal Nutritional Problem in the Himalayan Women", *Man in India* : 83(1&2) 29-48.

Pant, B.R., (in Press, b), "Housing and Environmental Sanitation Pattern in the Himalayan Village," *The Geographical Review of India,* Kolkata.

Pant, B.R., (in Press, c), Demographic Profile of Indian Himalya, *HIMVIKAS Journal* of GBPIHED, Almora.

Pant, B.R., (communicated), Environmental Degradation and Demographic Structure in Indian Himalaya, *The Indonesian Journal of Geography,* Indonesia.

Pant, B.R., and D.S. Jalal, (1991a), "State of Nutrition in Kotadun, Lesser Himalaya," *Annals of the NAGI,* 11(2): 64-67.

Pant, B.R., and D.S. Jalal, (1991b), "Nutrition Deficiency Disease in Indian Central Himalaya," *The Geographer.* 38(1) : 230-41.

Pant, B.R., and D.S. Jalal, (1996), "Environmental Hazards in Central Himalaya– A Case Study" in R.B. Singh (ed.), Research in Geography, *Disasters and Environment, Monitoring and Forecasting,* A.P.H. Publication, New Delhi, Vol ll: 291-298.

Papola, T.S., (2000), "Contradiction in Development of Uttarakhand: Need for Region-Specific and Autonomous Planning Framework," In M.C. Sati and S.P. Sati (eds.), *Uttarakhand Statehood: Dimensions of Development,* Indus Publishing Company, New Delhi, 56-66.

Prentice, Ann, (1998), Calcium Requirements in Pregnancy and Lactation, *NFI Bulletin,* 19(2): 1-5.

Qureshi, M.H. and S. Kumar, (1996), "Housing and Sanitation in Rural Areas: A Micro-Level Analysis," *The Indian Geographical Journal,* 71(2): 81-93.

Ramachandran, P., (1989a), "Nutrition in Pregnancy," In C. Gopalan and Kaur (eds.), *Women and Nutrition in India,* NFI Special Publication, Series 5: 153-193.

Ramachandran, P., (1989b), "Lactation – Nutrition – Fertility Interaction," In Gopalan and S. Kaur (eds.), *Women and Nutrition in India,* NFI Special Publication, Series 5: 194-223.

Ramachandran, P., (1996), Vitamin a Supplementation in Pregnancy and Lactation, *NFI Bulletin,* 74(4): 6-8.

Ramtora, K.C., (1989), "Female Work Participation: A Geographical Perspective with Special Reference to Marathwada," *The Indian Geographical Journal,* 64(1): 80-87.

Ramtora, K.C., (1995), Socio-Economic Status of Women in Maharastra: A Geographical Perspective, *The Indian Geographical Journal*, 70(2): 98-103.

Rao, B.S.N., (1989), Nutrient Requirement and RDA of Girls and Women in India. In C. Gopalan and S. Kaur (eds.), *Women and Nutrition in India*, NFI Special Publication Series 5 : 63-107.

Rao, B.S.N., (1996), "Bioavailability of b-Carotene Form Plant Foods," *NFI Bulletin* 17(4): 1-5.

Reiger, H.C., (1981), "Man verses Mountain: The Destruction of the Himalayan Ecosystem," In J.S. Lall and A.D. Moddie (eds.), *Himalaya: Aspects of Change*, Oxford Unipress, New Delhi, 351-376.

Sachdev, H.P.S., (1997), "Nutritional Status of Children and Women in India: Recent Trends," *NFI Billetin*, 18(3): 1-5.

Salaff, J., (1976), "Status of Unmaried Hong Women and the Social Factors Contributing to Their Delayed Marriage," *Population Studies*, 30(3): 391-412.

Samuel, L.K. and P.S.S. Rao, (1992), "Socio-Economic Differentials in Mothers at Risk Based on Pre-Pregnancy Weights and Heights," *Indian Journal of Medical Research*, 96: 159-167.

Santhanan, M., (1989), "Community Participation and Rural Water Supply and Sanitation Programme," *Social Change*, 19(1): 53-58.

Shah, S.L., (1982), "Ecological Degradation and Future of Agriculture in the Himalaya," *Indian Journal of Agricultural Economics*, 37(1): 1-22. Reprinted in B.R. Pant and M.C. Pant, (eds.), (1995), *Glimpses of Central Himalaya*, Radha Publications, New Delhi, 422-499.

Simpson, J.W., R.W. Lawless and A.C. Mitchell, (1975), "Responsibility of the Obsterician to the Fetus 11," *Influence of Pregnancy Weight and Pregnancy Weight Gain on Birth Weight*, Obstet, Gyncol, 45: 481-487.

Singh J.S. and A.K. Saxena, (1980), Analysis of Forest Grazing and Vegetation in Parts of Kumaun Himalaya, *Indian Journal of Range Management,* 1(1) : 13-32.

Singh J.S., U. Pandey and A.K. Tiwari, (1984), "Man and Forests: A Central Himalayan Case Study," *Ambio,* 13(2) 80-87.

Sood, A.K. and B.K. Nagla, (1999), "Social Ceremonies, Indigenous and Cultural Practices Affecting Maternal and Child Health in Rural Area of Haryana," *Region, Health and Health Care,* 4(2): 1-5.

Srikantia, S.G., (1989), "Pattern of Growth and Development of Indian Girls and Body Size of Adult Indian Women," In C. Gopalan and S. Kaur (eds.), *Women and Nutrition in India,* NFI Special Publication, Series 5: 108-152.

Tripathi, A.M., D.K. Agrawal, K.N. Agrawal, R.R. Devi and S. Cherian, (1987), "Nutrition Status of Rural Pregnant Women and Fetal Outcome," *Indian Pediatrics,* 24: 703-712.

Valdiya, K.S., (1980), "Stratigraphic Scheme of the Sedimentary Units of the Kumaun Lesser Himalaya," In K.S. Valdiya and S.B. Bhatia (eds.), *Stratigraphy and Correlation of Lesser Himalayan Formations,* HPC, Delhi, 7-48.

Valdiya, K.S., (1985), "Accelerated Erosion and Landsides Prone Zone in the Central Himalayan Region," In J.S. Singh (ed.), *Environmental Regeneration in Himalaya: Concepts and Strategies,* CHEA & Gyanodaya Prakashan, Nainital, 12-38.

Valdiya K.S., (1987), *Environmental Geology: Indian Context T.M.H.,* New Delhi, 583p.

Valdiya, K.S., (1988), "Geology of Kumaun: An Outline," In K.S. Valdiya (ed.), *Kumaun: Land and People,* Gyanodaya Prakashan, Nainital, 37-72.

Valdiya K.S., (1992), "The Uttarkashi Earthquake of 20th October: Implications and Lessons," *Current Science 61(12),* 25 December: 801-803.

Valdiya K.S. and S.K. Bartarya, (1991), "Hydrological Studies of Springs in the Catchment of Gaula River, Kumaun Lesser Himalaya, India," *Mountain Research and Development,* 11(3): 239-258.

Vir, S.C., and A.K. Nigam, (2001), Nutrition Status of Children in Uttar Predesh, *NFI Bulletin,* 22(1): 4-6.

Wong, O.M.H., (1999), Indicators of Women's Social Status as Determinants of the Marital Timing of Women in Hong Kong, *Asian Profile,* 27(5): 389-400.

Wong, Thomas W.P., (1995), "Women and Work: Opportunities and Experiences," In Veronica Pearson and Benjamin K.P. Leung (eds.), *Women in Hong Kong,* Hong Kong, Oxford University Press, 47-73.

INDEX